THE ART THERAPISTS' PRIMER

ABOUT THE EDITORS

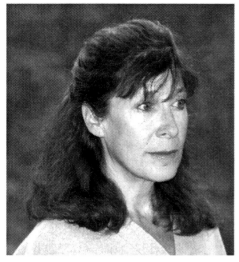

Photo by Nancy Bachrach.

Dr. Ellen G. Horovitz, Ph.D., ATR-BC, LCAT, RYT is Professor/Director of Graduate Art Therapy and the Art Therapy Clinic at Nazareth College of Rochester. She has had over thirty years of experience with myriad patient populations and specializes in family art therapy with the Deaf. Dr. Horovitz currently is in private practice and is the author of numerous articles, book chapters and the following books: *Spiritual Art Therapy: An Alternate Path; A Leap of Faith: The Call to Art; Art Therapy As Witness: A Sacred Guide;* and *Visually Speaking: Art Therapy and the Deaf.* As well, Dr. Horovitz has directed and produced ten films available in DVD format (Dr. Horovitz's films are available through www.arttxfilms.com). She is past President Elect of the American Art Therapy Association (AATA), currently serves as a Board Director for the Society for the Arts in Healthcare (www.theSAH.org), and is Media Editor for the forthcoming Society for the Arts in Healthcare journal, *Arts and Health: Research, Policy and Practice.* She recently completed a rigorous seven-month, 200+ hour Iyengar Yoga Essential Teacher Training under the renowned Francois Raoult, MS. Dr. Horovitz incorporates Yoga Therapy at her Art Therapy Clinic at Nazareth College of Rochester.

Sarah L. Eksten, MS, ATR received her Masters of Science in Creative Arts Therapy from Nazareth College in Rochester, New York. She also completed her undergraduate in Psychology at Nazareth College of Rochester. Sarah has experience working with children described as "at-risk" at the Mt. Hope Family Center, University of Rochester's Strong Memorial Hospital Psychiatric Department, and has also worked with the developmentally disabled at the Arc of Monroe's Community Art Connection. Currently, she works as an Art Therapist at Continuing Developmental Services (CDS), and the Mental Health Coalition (MHC) of the Mental Health Association in Rochester, NY.

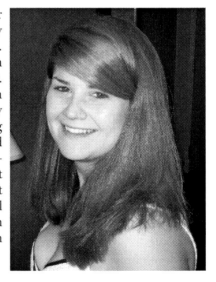

THE ART THERAPISTS' PRIMER

A Clinical Guide to Writing Assessments, Diagnosis, and Treatment

Edited by

ELLEN G. HOROVITZ, Ph.D., ATR-BC, LCAT, RYT

and

SARAH L. EKSTEN, MS, ATR

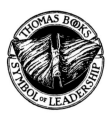

CHARLES C THOMAS • PUBLISHER, LTD.
Springfield • Illinois • U.S.A.

Published and Distributed Throughout the World by

CHARLES C THOMAS • PUBLISHER, LTD.
2600 South First Street
Springfield, Illinois 62704

© 2009 by CHARLES C THOMAS • PUBLISHER, LTD.

ISBN 978-0-398-07840-9 (hard)
ISBN 978-0-398-07841-6 (paper)

Library of Congress Catalog Card Number: 2008035727

Printed in the United States of America
SM-R-3

Library of Congress Cataloging-in-Publication Data

The art therapists' primer : a clinical guide to writing assessments, diagnosis,
and treatment / edited by Ellen G. Horovitz and Sarah L. Eksten.
    p. ; cm.
Includes bibliographical references and indexes.
ISBN 978-0-398-07840-9 (hard) -- ISBN 978-0-398-07841-6 (pbk.)
1. Art therapy. I. Horovitz, Ellen G. II. Eksten, Sarah L., 1981-
[DNLM: 1. Art Therapy--methods--Case Reports. WM 450.5.A8 A783863
2009]
RC489.A7A766 2009
616.89'1656--dc22

                                                                2008035727

*For my mother, Maida Pearl Shaw Horovitz, a mensch in action,
whose assessment of living life sustains my judgment and evaluation
of all things pivotal.*

E.G.H.

*To my parents, Larry and Clara Eksten, who have inspired me
to dream large and live freely to reach my highest potential.*

S.L.E.

CONTRIBUTORS

James Albertson, MS received his Masters of Science in Creative Arts Therapy from Nazareth College of Rochester in May, 2008. James was the recipient of the 2008 Alumni Award at Nazareth College of Rochester. James facilitated art therapy workshops at the Annual World Children's Art Festival in Washington, D.C. and participated in an international internship experience conducting art therapy in Tanzania, East Africa. Prior to his enrollment in the Creative Arts Therapy program at Nazareth College, James served as a United States Peace Corps Volunteer in Niger, West Africa and subsequently, provided extensive consulting services for the Carter Center, Inc. in Ghana and Mali. He is currently employed by the Carter Institute and is working as a primary therapist in Sudan, Africa.

Jacob M. Atkinson, MS is currently working as an Art Therapist/Clinical Case Manager for the Center for Psychosocial Development in Anchorage, Alaska. He recently graduated with his Masters of Science in Creative Art Therapies at Nazareth College in Rochester, New York. Jacob completed his undergraduate work at Utah State University, where he received his Bachelors of Fine Art with an emphasis in printmaking. Jacob also co-authored a chapter with Dr. Ellen Horovitz in her book (2007) *Visually Speaking: Art Therapy and the Deaf.*

Donna J. Betts, Ph.D., ATR-BC received a Bachelor of Fine Arts from the Nova Scotia College of Art & Design, a Master of Arts in Art Therapy from the George Washington University in 1999, and a PhD in Art Education with a specialization in Art Therapy from the Florida State University in 2005. Dr. Betts is currently a Director on the Art Therapy Credentials Board (ATCB). She served on the Board of Directors of the American Art Therapy Association (AATA) from 2002–2004. Presently, she is an adjunct professor in the art therapy department at FSU and provides art therapy to people who have eating disorders in Tallahassee, FL. Dr. Betts is the Recording Secretary and Virtual Assistant for the National Coalition of Creative Arts Therapies Associations (www.nccata.org), and serves on the Editorial Board of *The Arts in Psychotherapy* journal and is also the author of *Creative Art Therapies Approaches in Adoption and Foster Care: Contemporary Strategies for Working with Individuals and Families.*

Day Butcher, MS received her Masters of Science in Art Therapy from Nazareth College of Rochester in May, 2008. Ms. Butcher graduated from Roberts Wesleyan College, Rochester, New York with a Bachelor of Science in Art Education in May, 2003. She most recently participated in a three-week internship in Tanzania, East Africa. She currently is employed at the Center for Youth Services in the Runaway and Homeless Division in the Emergency Shelter in Rochester, NY.

Jen DeRoller, MS received her Masters of Science in Art Therapy from Nazareth College of Rochester in May, 2008. She also completed her undergraduate in Psychology at Nazareth College of Rochester. She currently is employed as a functional family therapist through the Cayuga Home for Children, Ithaca, NY.

Sarah L. Eksten, MS, ATR received her Masters of Science in Creative Arts Therapy from Nazareth College in Rochester, New York. She also completed her undergraduate in Psychology at Nazareth College of Rochester. Sarah has experience working with children described as "at-risk" at the Mt. Hope Family Center, University of Rochester's Strong Memorial Hospital Psychiatric Department, and has also worked with the developmentally disabled at the Arc of Monroe's Community Art Connection. Currently, she works as an Art Therapist at Continuing Developmental Services (CDS), and the Mental Health Coalition (MHC) of the Mental Health Association in Rochester, NY.

Ellen G. Horovitz, Ph.D., ATR-BC, LCAT, RYT is Professor/Director of Graduate Art Therapy and the Art Therapy Clinic at Nazareth College of Rochester. She has had over 30 years of experience with myriad patient populations and specializes in family art therapy with the Deaf. Dr. Horovitz currently is in private practice and is the author of numerous articles, book chapters and the following books: *Spiritual Art Therapy: An Alternate Path; A Leap of Faith: The Call to Art; Art Therapy As Witness: A Sacred Guide* and *Visually Speaking: Art Therapy and the Deaf.* As well, Dr. Horovitz has directed and produced ten films available in DVD format (Dr. Horovitz's films are available through www.arttxfilms.com). She is past President Elect of the American Art Therapy Association (AATA) and currently serves as a Board Director for the Society for the Arts in Healthcare (www.theSAH.org) and is Media Editor for the forthcoming Society for the Arts in Healthcare journal, *Arts and Health: Research, Policy and Practice.* She recently completed a rigorous seven-month, 200+ hour Iyengar Yoga Essential Teacher Training under the renowned Francois Raoult, MS. Dr. Horovitz incorporates Yoga Therapy at her Art Therapy Clinic at Nazareth College of Rochester.

Jordan M. Kroll, MS received his Masters of Science in Creative Arts Therapy from Nazareth College of Rochester in May, 2008. He is a worship artist and musician whose career will be dedicated to using the creative arts to facilitate spiritual healing and exploration. During his graduate education at Nazareth College of Rochester, NY, Jordan worked with developmentally disabled adults, children of high-stress environments, and adolescent and adult substance abusers. Jordan was recently named recipient of the Art Therapy Program's Academic Excellence

Award, and is currently doing missionary work in China, where he will be employing the spiritual language of visual art.

Barbara Murak, MS received her Masters of Science in Art Therapy from Nazareth College of Rochester in May, 2008. She has been a studio fiber artist for over 35 years, has exhibited her work in juried exhibitions both nationally and internationally, with work in public and private collections in the United States as well as in nine countries. Barbara's work has been featured in several journal publications, and she is a current member of the Surface Design Association, Buffalo Society of Artists, and the Fibre Design Forum.

Julie Riley, MS received her Masters of Science in Creative Arts Therapy from Nazareth College of Rochester in May, 2008. She also earned a BFA (2004) in Visual Media from Rochester Institute of Technology. Julie also explored her interest in cross-cultural trends by co-leading art therapy programs at the International Child Art Foundation's World Child Art Festival in 2007 and participating in an international internship in Tanzania, Africa in August, 2007 working with adolescent detainees. Currently, she is establishing an art therapy career in Houston, Texas.

Rachel N. Sikorski, MS, ATR is a graduate of the Creative Arts Therapy Program at Nazareth College in Rochester, New York and holds a Bachelor of Arts degree in Psychology, Art History, and German from Canisius College in Buffalo, New York. Currently, Rachel works at Gateway-Longview Lynde School in Williamsville, New York, a facility that serves youth with emotional and behavioral problems in both day treatment and residential education programs. Rachel is the primary art therapist for the residential C.A.B. (Changing Attitudes and Behaviors) Program, a critical care program in which youth with typically more aggressive and sexual acting-out behaviors receive a higher level of therapeutic treatment in a structured, self-contained setting.

Luke M. Sworts is currently a Research Assistant at the University of Rochester Medical Center where he is working on a NIMH-funded grant evaluating the efficacy of a school-based intervention program. He earned his BS from SUNY Geneseo where he majored in Psychology and Art Studio and is currently enrolled in the Creative Arts Therapy Graduate program at Nazareth College of Rochester. Luke's current clinical experience is with emotionally and behaviorally challenged youth. He has been included on several research publications and plans to pursue doctorate-level work related to his interests in art therapy and urban adolescents.

Maria Selman Pinto is a current graduate student at the MS Creative Arts Therapy program at Nazareth College of Rochester. She is from Santiago, Chile and has already completed a postgraduate specialization in Art Therapy. In her home country, she has had experience working with different populations, such as adults with cancer, abused children, and adolescents with mental disabilities. In addition, she is a founder member and past President and board of director of the Chilean Art Therapy Association.

PREFACE ON HOW TO USE THIS BOOK

You know how you get software and bundled in it is this small text file that says something like "Read This First"? Well, that's what I am hoping you will do before heading straight into the chapters. The reason is threefold: (1) if you are an educator you will want to know how to use this manual as a teaching tool; (2) it will save you some time in case you are an experienced clinician and merely want to flip around to gather what is pertinent to your practice; and (3) if you are new to the field (a student or even a seasoned graduate), it will afford you the armament to write up clinically-based reports that include assessments, objectives, modalities, goals, summaries, and termination reports. As well, the Appendices (A-G), provide you with a wealth of information and forms to use in your practice.

But bear with me for a moment, because the history of this book's birth represents a little over 25 years of my life as an educator. Around the early '90s, I developed a required textbook (which was published by Nazareth College in Rochester, NY) so that students would have a manual for (ATR 522 & ATR 523) my Assessment, Diagnosis and Counseling I and II, year-long class. As luck would have it, one day I found myself sitting on a tram next to my dear colleague, Dr. Rawley Silver, HLM, ATR-BC, on the way to an American Art Therapy Association (AATA) conference. Rawley was flipping through my treatise called the *Art Therapy Program Textbook,* (Horovitz, 1995), which every incoming student received and was required to read before entering Day 1 of classes. Suddenly, she turned to me and adamantly demanded, "You must make this available for purchase! Everyone in the field would benefit. Do it!!" (Mind you, this approximately 200-page text, aptly called the "Bible" by my students, was not for sale to anyone outside of my art therapy program.) But a strange thing happened: my students kept graduating and getting work, and more often than not as primary therapists. I slowly figured out that this was due not only to the medically-based training that the students received but more importantly, because they were able to *transliterate* their findings to a medical, educational, and/or clinical team. The "Bible" *(Art Therapy Program Textbook)* had secured them with the necessary armament to communicate their findings in a cogent manner. They could *walk the walk* but more significantly, they could *talk the talk.* So I knew that Rawley was right: it was time to share my main cooking ingredient (informed treatment) with others.

So after 25 some-odd years of educating, I decided to ask my recent students who had turned in A or A+ papers if they wanted to publish their samples in this (now) publicly available opus. And I decided to enlist one of my former students, Sarah Eksten, MS, ATR, to co-edit this opus with me. It was a win-win for everyone. My students got published (some even before graduating) and art therapists would be able to use my formula to cultivate a clinical recipe guaranteed to offer them acceptance in a scientific community, thus elevating the Art Therapy field.

So in a nutshell, that's the game plan in this book. All chapters of assessments (Chapters 1–10) walk the reader through the history of the actual assessment tool and how to administer it. Those chapters offer several case samples for the reader to purview so that he or she might be able to glean not only how to administer the test but also how one should write-up the results for dissemination to other clinicians.

So now let me tell you how it's organized:

- Chapter 1 – Gathering Client Information and Constructing a Genogram: This is the first step in creating a cogent treatment plan. The reader learns how to create a genogram (literally a visual map of a client's family system) and the importance of understanding the transitional conflicts handed down from generation to generation. This is Step 1 in understanding the identified patient (IP) as a product of his environmental family system, from the micro to the macro-system. Additionally, this construct can include psychological scores (intelligence quotient scores such as a WISC-R), strengths and weaknesses, DSM IV-TR (soon to be DSM V-TR) information from the attending psychiatrist, and visual symbols that all clinicians can code and understand. As well, a chronological timeline is created which maps out any nodal events that have affected the IP's history. It is important to note that *Appendix A* has the genograms of every client used throughout this book in the varying chapters. Tab it so you can flip to it as you read the various assessments in each chapter.
- Chapter 2 – The Art Therapy Dream Assessment (ATDA): This simple assessment was developed (Horowitz, 1999) to offer insight into objectives and treatment goals to move the client towards resolve of unresolved emotional conflicts while contemporaneously offering perception, information, and direction to the clinician. This tool cuts through the tangled undercurrents of dream information that often bubbles to the conscious surface in an array of confusing metaphors, symbols, and personalities. The magical sword yielded by the art therapist is the result of mirroring back the client's words through empathic reading and simultaneous viewing of the nonverbal (i.e., artistic response to the dream). Samples abound from varying pathologies offering the reader a rich mixture of case studies.
- Chapter 3 – Belief Art Therapy Assessment (BATA): When indicated, the BATA is deployed when a client questions his or her belief system and/or brings up issues of faith (wavering or not). (However, it should be underscored that one should employ the BATA **only** when warranted. The reason is that when florid, psychotic thinking is present, conducting the test in its entirety can in fact exacerbate this condition, plaguing emotionally disturbed individuals.) In this chapter, the reader again gets a full sense of not only how to conduct this assessment but how to view the findings for treatment and resolve of belief system issues.

- Chapter 4 – Bender-Gestalt II: The new calibration system involved in the revision of the Bender-Gestalt II walks the reader through a procedure that systematically ranks original and new test cards along a continuum of difficulty. Beyond the Copy Test, the new version now employs a Recall Test, and Global Scoring System. Additionally, instruction on the new Motor and Perception test is added with several cases of varying pathology. These samples offer the administrant a scientific and empirical test that reviews cognitive, perceptual, neurological, and emotive functioning.

- Chapter 5 – Cognitive Art Therapy Assessment (CATA): This assessment tool is guised as an open-ended studio activity and thus little to no stress is involved on the subject's part. Since it does not feel like a "test" since the directive is open-ended, the client is virtually unaware that his or her response can later be measured for cognitive and developmental change on pretest/posttest measure when utilizing Lowenfeld and Brittain's (1975) developmental scoring system (based on norms for Art Education) or using Horovitz's Adult, Artistic or Brain Injured Stages and scoring system (Horovitz, 2002). Indeed, these artistic developmental stages offer a "snapshot" for the art therapist when beginning treatment planning and preparing to use two and three-dimensional media to facilitate emotional, physical, cognitive, and spiritual recovery. Again full instructions on administration follow with several case vignettes.

- Chapter 6 – Face Stimulus Assessment (FSA): In this chapter Donna Betts, author of the FSA, defines the history, use of this assessment, and current research indications. Following, the chapter presents two case studies using the FSA, one with a traumatic brain-injured client. For both of these cases, the informal rating procedure from the FSA Guidelines (Betts, 2008) was used to formulate possible interpretations of the drawings.

- Chapter 7 – House-Tree-Person Test (HTP): The subtests of the HTP are saturated with symbolic, emotional, and ideational experiences linked to personality development; therefore, the drawings of these images drive projection of the drawer. Developmentally, the favorite drawing object of young children has been touted as the human figure, followed by the house, and then the tree. While the authors will not cover all of the specific interpretations of the HTP, the editors redirect the reader to the Hammer (1980) text for an in-depth review of these variables. Administration of the subtests is reviewed and presentation of various case samples follow.

- Chapter 8 – Kinetic Family Drawing (KFD): As a clinician for over 30 years, Horovitz (2002, 2005, 2007) has found the KFD to be the single most important projective tool in her arsenal. This simple projective task can elicit information that recreates all the transitional conflicts handed down from generation to generation (as gleaned from the IP genogram). While analysis of the KFD symbols are expressed in great detail in Burns and Kaufman's (1972) opus, the authors again point the reader back to that book in order to offer the reader a more detailed account of the symbolic meanings of barriers, competition, action items, compartmentalization, and so forth. Several case samples follow the historical review, administration of this instrument, and review of the analysis and grid sheets, which accompany this battery.

- Chapter 9 – Person Picking an Apple from a Tree (PPAT): The manual, administration, and history of Gantt & Tabone's instrument, the PPAT (including the Formal Elements Art Therapy Scale (FEATS) as the rating instrument for the assessment), are reviewed with a method for deciphering and understanding the nonsymbolic aspects of art. Formulation of the structural characteristics and diagnosis of the IP's clinical state is highlighted as well as the primary focus of the instrument, to witness *how* people drew as opposed to hone in on *what* they drew. As well, "pattern matching" that is to distinguish the differences between the four classic Axis I disorders (major depression, schizophrenia, organic mental disorders, and bipolar disorder) as correlated with the FEATS is presented along with the review of this instrument via several case studies.
- Chapter 10 – Silver Drawing Test (SDT): In the review of the SDT, the assessment of three concepts fundamental to mathematics and reading are highlighted in the subtests of this battery, which allows for pretest and posttest reviews of the IP. Silver's work is based on Jean Piaget (1967, 1970), who remains famous for his work in conservation and spatial concepts. This short, easy-to-administer battery can be readily used when working with clients, even those who have short attention spans. Again several vignettes are offered for the reader and all aspects of the test (including scoring system and emotive scales – based on empirically valid studies) are covered in this review.
- Chapter 11 – From Africa to America: Art Assessments with a Refugee in Resettlement: Assessing the mental health of refugees in resettlement is a complex process that is often convoluted by language and intercultural barriers (Misra, Connolly, & Majeed, 2006; Savin, Seymour, Littleford, & Giese, 2005). In this chapter, James (Jim) Albertson conducted one of the most thorough assessments that ever passed before Horovitz in her year-long assessment class. Jim had been privy to working with this client throughout the semester and thus was able to draw significant conclusions based on the IP's genogram, timeline, and cultural diversity. Six art-based assessments were conducted with this adult refugee from Burundi, Africa during his eight months of resettlement in Rochester, NY. Jim's excellent synopsis presents a very thorough review of many of the assessments presented within this book and offers the reader a thorough sample of an art therapy assessment combining various batteries.
- Chapter 12 – Assessments, Treatment, Termination Summaries and Internet-Based Referrals: In this final chapter, Horovitz presents varying assessments and treatment samples that one might see when working on an interdisciplinary team or as a private practitioner. Abbreviated assessments, a creative arts therapy termination summary, a long-term Art Therapy Termination summary (complete with objectives), and a sample from an Internet-based referral are amongst the highlights of this chapter. These are offered as illustrations of what a practitioner (neophyte or experienced) might bump up against in career and private practice. Appendices C thru G are filled with some of the various forms that highlight this important culminating chapter.

In conclusion, while *all* the assessments that are currently available to art therapy practitioners are *not* covered in this treatise, what is offered is a systematic review of the assessments outlined above. These assessments were *chosen* because of their *ease* in administration as well as the information procured for the practitioner. The SDT and Bender-Gestalt II have been empirically tested and both can be used for pretest and posttest purposes. The CATA was chosen specifically since it is guised as an open-ended, non-directive battery, thus eliminating stress (Horovitz & Schulze, 2008). As well, the CATA can also be used for pretest and posttest purposes, and has been submitted for empirical testing as part of an NIH-funded pilot study.

Additionally, the practitioner is offered sample formats, legends and abbreviations of clinical and psychiatric terms, guidelines for recordable significant events, instructions on writing-up objectives, modalities, and treatment goals as well as training on composing progress versus process notes.

It is hoped that this book will serve as a companion guide for every art therapist in creating clinical reports on patients to aid their trajectory towards wellness, recovery and above all, health.

E.G.H.

ACKNOWLEDGMENTS

Books take time and constant seasoning until they are baked, just like a good meal. But this treatise has been a wholly different order since the concoction being stirred was not only my words and work, but also that of many of my students who contributed to the chapters herein. For it is my students that I wish to thank and acknowledge. As Jacob Bronoski said, *"It is important that students bring a certain ragamuffin barefoot irreverence to their studies. They are here . . . to question it."*

Yet, categorically, I need to thank some very important people who continue to sustain me and have been in my life for the long haul: my immediate family and friends: Dr. Nancy Bachrach, Dr. Len Horovitz, Orin Wechsberg, Valerie Saalbach, Maida Horovitz, Kaitlyn Leah Darby, Bryan James Darby, and *specifically* my closest colleagues and "partners in crime", Lori Houlihan Higgins, ATR-BC, LCAT and Dr. William D. Schulze. As well, I wish to wholeheartedly thank my editor at Charles C Thomas, Claire Slagle, who has fine-tuned all my books. Claire, as always, thank you for all your hard work. And, of course, Michael Thomas for your vision and all your support over the years.

Above all, I wish to thank my patients, whose stories and whose hearts I have held and entwined with mine, as we worked towards a trajectory of wellness. Thank you for giving meaning to my life.

E.G.H.

As this is my first book as a published author, I want to thank Dr. Horovitz, my professor and mentor who provided me with this opportunity. I also want to thank my colleagues who patiently worked with me on this book.

S.L.E.

CONTENTS

FIGURES

COLOR PLATES

THE ART THERAPISTS' PRIMER

Chapter 1

GATHERING CLIENT INFORMATION AND CONSTRUCTING A GENOGRAM

In completing an art therapy assessment on a client, you will first need to create a genogram. A genogram is a three-generation (minimum) visual map of an identified patient's (IP) family system. Additionally, this construct can include psychological scores (intelligence quotient scores such as a WISC-R), strengths and weaknesses, DSM IV-TR (soon to be DSM V-TR) information from the attending psychiatrist, and visual symbols that help you and your supervisor track conflicts handed down from generation to generation. As well, a chronological time-line is created which maps out any nodal events that have affected the patient's history. Generally, these days the instructions are so simple that they can even be found on the Internet: http://sfhelp.org/03/geno1.htm

Indeed here are the instructions from that page:

Symbol Conventions

Here are some "standard" symbols to use:

- Use 3/4" circles for females, and squares for males. Crosshatch or color these for extra-important people (important to whom?). Use dashed circles and squares, or slashed or "X'd" symbols, to represent dead, missing, or psychologically-detached people;
- Horizontal solid lines show legal marriages, and dashed lines to show committed unmarried primary relationships, and important friendships, dependencies, hero/ines, and supporters. A horizontal line with a $--//--$ or $--X--$ can indicate a psychological or legal divorce;
- Vertical or slanted solid lines show genetic connections. Dashed slanted lines can show adoptions, foster parents, or other special adult-child rela-

3

tionships. Option – use double, triple, or colored lines to indicate the importance or relative strength of the connection between two people;

- Zigzag, double, or wavy lines can symbolize strong emotional, legal, financial, or other kinds of current relationship connections, including lust, grief, anger, fear, and "hatred." If helpful, add symbols like "+" and "–" to show friendship, love, hostility, and/or fear;
- Draw an "X" through a circle or square to indicate death;
- Include names, dates, pets, extra-important current friends, sponsors, or authorities, major illnesses and disabilities, addictions, arrows for child visitations, and any other symbolic or text information that adds clarity and meaning to your map.

In the editors' opinion, the *best* source for truly understanding this book was recently re-edited by McGoldrick, Gerson, & Petry (2008). This book gives you numerous samples and in depth cases to understand the importance of this visual map as well as more complex samples such as miscarriage, suicide, and other nodal events that are either effecting the IP (identified patient) and/or family system.

Again, it is important to note that we do not, by any means, live in isolation and we are affected by not only our family system (thus making the term

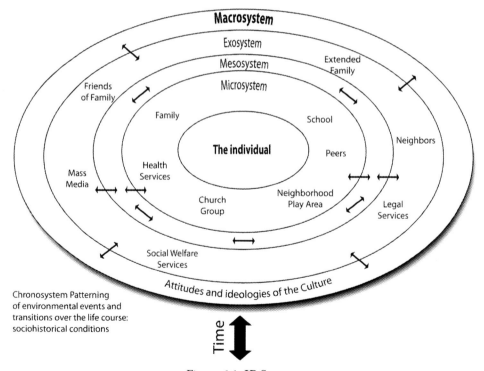

Figure 1.1. IP System.

IP almost contradictory); but we are also affected by an even larger system that impacts are entire personality including the macrosystem such as above.

All of these factors contribute to who we are and what we become as individual players within our society. So while the reader might be mapping the IP's genogramatic system, it is paramount to note that we not only do not operate in isolation, but also, the therapist needs to work from a family system's perspective, even if the family is not present. This can be done through artwork, empty chairs, and then some. So as the reader will see, the thrust of this book views the individual through the eyes of the collective whole and all of its influence.

When beginning to understand this concept, as a professor and author, Horovitz always makes the first assignment in her assessment class for each student to create a three-generation genogram of him or herself. The reason is multifaceted: (a) it initiates the student's understanding of exactly how these factors above contribute to his or her shaping as a human being operating in this world; (b) it sets the stage for the student to be able to ask the proper questions of clients (or intake workers) to construct a genogram to understand that client's genogramatic system; and (c) most importantly, it allows the student to hold onto his or her own genogram and take a good hard look at exactly how the psychosocial issues of his or her family system impact both the transference and countertransference with each individual case. Horovitz also encourages each student to then share this genogram in the confidential setting of academic supervision in order to extract maximum supervision. After over 30 years of teaching, this has proven to be an enormous asset to student understanding and processes.

Within the following pages, the reader will find some examples at collecting behavioral observations, psychosocial indicators, and constructing a genogram with timeline.

Identified Patient: S

DOB: 2000

CA: 6 years old

Testing Dates: February 26, 2006; March 6, 2006; March 27, 2006

Administrant: Jacob Atkinson

Assessments Administered: CATA, PPAT, SDT

See Chapters 5, 9, and 10 respectively, for further examples regarding S.

Behavioral Observations

   S presents herself as an intelligent, well-groomed six-year-old, whose physical size is closer to that of a four-year-old. S's size is a result of her medically restricted diet of fruits and vegetables due to Eosinophilic Gastroenteritis. S's mother is Deaf and her father is hard of hearing, requiring S to learn and communicate by using both speech and sign language. S is friendly upon entering the clinic and even more so after her mother leaves.

History and Genogram

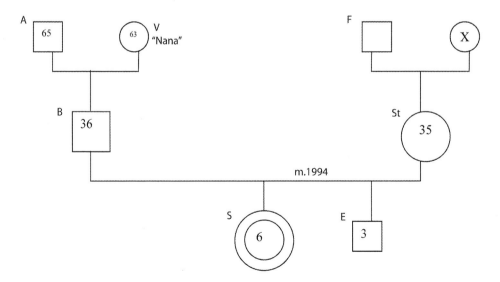

Figure 1.2. S's Genogram.

Timeline

- 1-year-old and becomes ill
- 3-year-old S is diagnosed with Eosinophilic Gastroenteritis (EG) which currently only allows her to eat selected fruits and vegetables
- Her disorder has caused her many surgeries and tests
- 6-year-old S becomes frustrated with food restrictions
- S spent over a month at the KKI hospital in Baltimore for EG in November, 2005
- Returned to Hospital for a weekend checkup in April, 2006
- Mother is Deaf
- Father is hard of hearing
- Both paternal grandparents are Deaf

Identified Patient: Nathan

CA: 26.9

DOB: April 5, 1979

Testing Date: April 2, 2006

Administrant: Sarah L. Eksten

Assessments Administered: ATDA, KFD, SDT

See Chapters 2, 8, and 10 respectively, for further examples regarding Nathan.

Psychosocial Indicators

Nathan is a 26-year-old Caucasian male who resides in a four-bedroom house with three other male roommates in Rochester, NY. He is in a long-term, committed relationship with his girlfriend, Jennifer, of 1.3 years. Nathan is currently pursuing his doctoral degree in Microsystems at Rochester Institute of Technology (RIT). In addition to attending school, he works at RIT as a research assistant. Nathan was the first born to Charlie and Jane in Baltimore, Maryland. His sister, Allison, was born two years later (see Genogram). Nathan moved to Rochester when he was 18 to attend RIT for his undergraduate degree in Microelectronic Engineering. Since then, he has resided in Rochester, except for one year when he worked in Belgium as a researcher.

Behavioral Observations

Nathan agreed to meet with the administrant. He presented himself as a well-groomed, attractive, cooperative individual, eager to complete the testing. He sat at the table patiently, pencil in hand, waiting for the instructions. Throughout the session, he gave meticulous attention to each art piece; although, it did not take him more than 15 minutes to complete any of the pictures. Before he announced he was complete with each picture, he would stop drawing, sit back in his chair, and look at his creation to make sure it was either complete, needed additions, or was to his liking. He would then look at the writer, turn the paper so that she could look at it from the correct angle, and wait patiently for questions. Nathan seemed a little tense when answering questions provided by the administrant, possibly because he wanted to make sure he provided the information she was looking for.

History and Genogram

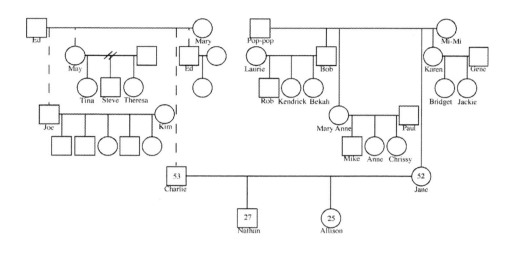

Figure 1.3. Nathan's Genogram.

Timeline

1979 – Nathan is born

1981 – Allison is born

1997 – Nathan attends RIT for undergraduate school

2002 – Nathan begins Ph.D. program

2003 – Nathan moves to Belgium for one year

2004 – Nathan returns from Belgium; starts dating Jennifer; starts back at RIT for Ph.D. program

Client: Pam

DOB: August 1954

CA: 52

Testing Dates: September 27, 2006; March 21, 2007; March 28, 2007

Administrant: Julie Riley

Tests Administered: BATA, FSA, SDT

See Chapters 3, 6, and 10 respectively, for further examples regarding Pam.

Psychosocial Indicators

Pam is a single, white, 52-year-old female. Currently she lives with five housemates who help compose Pam's support system: these also include friends at DayHab, PRALID staff, and her advocate (literacy volunteer). Her remaining family, consisting of two older sisters, lives in New York State although not in the Rochester vicinity. Pam suffered a traumatic brain injury (TBI) following a head-on collision motor vehicle accident (MVA) at the age of 16. Her boyfriend, the driver, died. Pam was in a coma for four months and received intensive medical attention and interventions. Between the time of the accident and 1986 her history is vague; but beginning in 1986 Pam rotated through several group homes in Connecticut until 1997 when she was moved to Rochester, NY as advocated by her social worker. In 2002, she was monitored for a possible breast tumor. Also in September of 2002, Pam began stating intentions of self harm and suicidal ideations; though this was concluded to be attention-seeking behavior, she was recommended for counseling. During counseling, it was concluded that Pam was having difficulties around issues of mourning and loss of her life prior to accident, death of her boyfriend, and her deceased parents.

Behavioral Observations

Pam has a vibrant sense of humor and keen intellectual ability; she likes mathematics and occasionally speaks French (her mother was French). She is very fashion conscious and makes efforts to "look good." She uses a wheelchair due to left hemiparesis and subsequently has suffered visual impairment. Her memory is primarily limited to proximity and events prior to the MVA. Her medical chart indicates that she occasionally struggles with distinguishing reality from imagination; but in art therapy sessions this writer has been privy to imaginative expression on several occasions during which Pam was oriented in reality.

History and Genogram

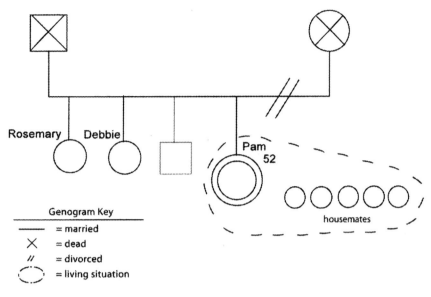

Figure 1.4. Pam's Genogram.

Timeline

8/54 – Born

1969 – Parents Divorce

11/70 – MVA; head-on collision, severe head injuries, brain trauma right side (left hemiparesis), comatose for 4 months, tracheotomy

Date unknown – Mother dies (heart attack)

4/86 – Admitted to Re-Entry Program at Golden Hill Health Care Center (Kingston, NY)

8/92 – Datahr ICF – Sweetcake Mountain group home (CT)

6/93 – Moved to Datahr ICF – Saw Mill group home (CT)
1/96 – Moved to Dorset Lane ICF group home (CT)

1997 – Moved to Rochester, NY

2002 – Monitored for possible breast tumor

9/2002 – Begins counseling due to statements of self harm and suicidal ideation

6/2006 – Referred to Nazareth Art Therapy Clinic

   * It is unclear as to when Pam's father died; but at some point after mom dies and before being transferred to Rochester, NY, notations in paperwork indicate he is deceased.

Chapter 2

ART THERAPY DREAM ASSESSMENT (ATDA)

MESSAGES DOWN UNDER

I have dreamt this dream every night since I can remember.
(Horovitz, 1999)

If a client said that to you, as Brett did to Horovitz (1999), would you have an assessment that allowed you to get at the meaning of what was affecting him or her? You could, with the ATDA (Horovitz, 1999). It's simple, easy and produces information that would not necessarily be available otherwise. It is also a very powerful tool in terms of jump-starting the therapeutic relationship.

Indeed, this simple assessment may offer insight into objectives and treatment goals to move the client towards resolve of unresolved emotional conflicts while contemporaneously offering perception, information, and direction. This tool cuts through the tangled undercurrents of dream information that often bubbles to the conscious surface in an array of confusing metaphors, symbols, and personalities. The magical sword yielded by the art therapist is the result of mirroring back the client's words through empathic reading and simultaneous viewing of the nonverbal (i.e., artistic response to the dream). It is in this mix that the dreamer can finally make sense of his or her unconscious deliberations and awaken to a conscious state aware of the contextual meaning and how these down-under messages may affect one's day-to-day operative relationships with others and life situations.

As will be seen from the samples below, the information produced through the written script literally funnels this dream information down to a manageable chignon, creating a headdress of clarity for the client and the therapist.

ADMINISTRATION OF THE ADTA

- Ask the client to choose a dream that has either reoccurred, happened recently, delighted or troubled him (or her). Then illustrate it in oil pastels, pastels, drawing media, paint, clay or other 3-dimensional material. Next, write a paragraph description of the dream. (N.B.: In order to funnel this down and get at the meat of the dream, the client is next asked to read the paragraph. The beauty in this assessment is the following: *read the written work back to the client.* The magic comes from the effect, rhythm, and tenor of the therapist's voice. The clients can actually hear the written paragraph differently when enunciated and effectively read by his or her therapist.)

- Next, the client then chooses a cluster of words that truly captures the essence of the dream. <u>Underline those words.</u> Client reads the cluster. Then the therapist *reads the cluster of words back* to the client.

- Then, the client *reduces* the cluster of words further and either (circles) the next words or <u>underlines them twice</u>. Then *read* the reduced underlined words back to the client.

- Next, ask the client to *reduce* the cluster to approximately 8 words that truly stand out. Then the therapist *reads the cluster of 8 words back* to the client.

- Finally, the client utilizes those 8 words and combines them into a single sentence. (Please note that articles such as "a," "the," "and," and so on can be used to create grammatical sentence structure. Moreover, the client can add endings such as "-ed" or "-ing" to words for the same structural purpose. It matters not how those 8 words are arranged so long as the client, not the therapist, administers the arrangement of the words in the sentence. The therapist can aid the client (if requested) regarding grammatical and syntax structure.) The client reads the sentence. Then the therapist *reads that back* to the client.

- This final process of writing a complete sentence, which sums up the experience, is what generally causes the "Ah-ha" phenomenon, thus allowing for insight not just into the artwork illustrating the client's dream, but also this exercise catapults the client towards deeper introspection on psychosocial, emotive issues that may plaque the client's progress and recovery. Horovitz (1999) aptly pointed this out in a fascinating case study on a young bipolar boy who had been severely beaten by his biological father. The dream was the result of this child's very realistic fear about his father's impending release from prison and the possibility that his father might abuse him again.

N.B.: Utilizing this process of the ATDA, Horovitz (1999) was able to help this aforementioned client look at the disparate parts of himself in the dream and thus enabled him to discuss not only his aggressive feelings (thus identifying with both the abuser and the victim), but also his own identification with the parts of himself that he wanted to "kill off." The focus of the treatment resulted from this activity and the client made great gains in the work ahead.

Examples of the ATDA are given.

Identified Patient: Holly

DOB: 1978

CA: 27

Testing Dates: April 2, 2006

Administrant: Jane C. Adams

Assessments Administered: ATDA, HTP, PPAT

See Chapters 7 and 9 for further examples regarding Holly.

Refer to Appendix A for Genogram, Timeline, Behavioral Observations, and Psychosocial Indicators.

The writer administered the ATDA to Holly with a directive to choose a dream (recurring or not, troubling or not), then to select materials and illustrate the dream. On completion of the illustration the writer and the client completed the written and verbal processes to arrive at a descriptive paragraph, a series of key words, and a sentence distilled from the combination (Horovitz, 1999).

Holly has had a recurring dream happening anywhere from once per month to twice per night for several years. In the dream, she plays the main role. There appear to be no other specifically remembered individuals in her dream such as family members. Holly's dream seems to escalate in intensity as she seeks to reach a goal or complete a task. She noted that it starts out as a normal dream; but as it progresses she is faced with a constant stream of obstacles. As her frustration grows she is even disturbed by intruders or onlookers at a point when she feels she most needs privacy. Her description of the dream further reinforces information apparent from Holly's House-Tree-Person (HTP) Assessment (see Chapter 7). Her search for privacy and her growing level of anxiety, when she is unable to find it, seem to be the major focus of her dream.

Sandy's Dream:

In my recurring dream, the premise is always the same. I have a goal or task to accomplish, but I come in contact with obstacle after obstacle, which ultimately prevents me from completing the task. The goal is always something very private, such as changing my clothes, going to the bathroom, or taking a shower. I start off in a normal dream, and the task will work itself in. From that point on, I'm on a mission to accomplish this goal. Just when I think I've found a private, safe place, something or someone will interfere. It may be intruding people, it may be onlookers,

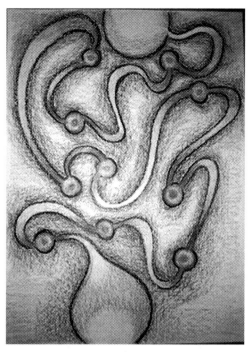

Figure 2.1. Sandy's ATDA Response. (For color version, see Plate 1, p. 109.)

it may be a bathroom stall that has no door or toilet paper, and so forth. Then I move on to try to find someplace else to finish my task, but another problem interferes. There's never any privacy, nothing works out as planned, <u>frustration</u> ensues, and the goal is left <u>unsatisfied</u>. The setting is different every time, but the problem is always essentially the same.

Cluster 1: Obstacle, Private, Task, Goal, Mission, Safe, Interfere, Problem, Frustration, Unsatisfied, Bathroom, Onlookers

Cluster 2: Obstacle, Private, Mission, Frustration, Bathroom, Unsatisfied, Interfere

Final Sentence: "I needed a private bathroom to complete my mission, but obstacle after obstacle interfered, leaving me unsatisfied and full of frustration."

Sandy chose these key words following our reading her paragraph. She then reduced her selection to the most essential. She completed the assessment by using the words in the second cluster to formulate a sentence describing the essence of her dream. Her choices further emphasize some of her HTP results (see Chapter 7). In addition, it appears that Holly remains in the Anal Stage of Psychosexual Development (Lowenfeld & Brittain, 1975). Her dream and assessment results illustrate Holly's focus on the attributes of this period (Stevenson, 1992). Holly's life experiences may have pro-hibited her exit from this stage and forced her to remain in the anal stage of development.

Conclusion

Holly possibly has issues and inner personal conflict, which may be creat-ing anxiety and frustration for her. All of her assessment results appear to indicate a set of unresolved issues. These seem to be related to her need for privacy and her struggle to cope with intimacy. Her drawings seem to indi-cate that she has achieved a measure of maturity visible in reaching Horovitz's (2002) Artistic Stage. Yet she remains stuck in Freud's Anal Stage of psychosexual development. She appears to be conflicted in her relation-ship with her family, both needing their attention and retreating from their presence.

Recommendations

To deal with her intimacy issues, the writer suggests a series of group art therapy sessions in order to develop the skills Holly might need to cope with and to succeed in family art therapy. The writer also recommends that Holly pursue a course of family art therapy.

Identified Patient: Nathan

CA: 26.9

DOB: April 5, 1979

Testing Date: April 2, 2006

Administrant: Sarah L. Eksten

Assessments Administered: ATDA, KFD, SDT

See Chapters 1, 8, and 10 for further examples regarding Nathan.

Refer to Appendix A for Genogram, Timeline, Behavioral Observations, and Psychosocial Indicators.

Nathan completed the Art Therapy Dream Assessment (ATDA). Although there were coloring media to work with, he decided to use pencil. Nathan described the dream in the paragraph that accompanied the picture:

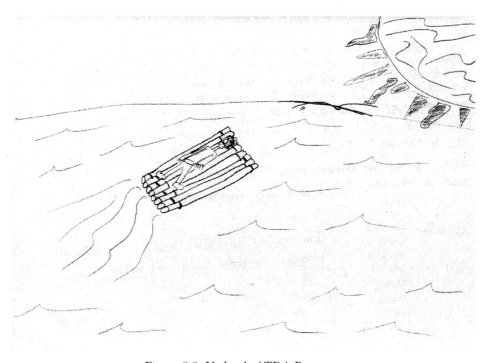

Figure 2.2. Nathan's ATDA Response.

> This is a reoccurring dream that I have. I'm stranded on a raft in the middle of the ocean. There is no land, no wind, no fresh water, no clouds; just the sun, the raft, the ocean, and me. In the dream I'm not panicking, just lonely, bored, and stuck on a raft. Sometimes I feel like the raft is sinking, but I just let it sink and not bother me. There aren't any sharks or fish; just me and the entire ocean. I usually just wait on the raft for a while and then I wake up.

Although he stated that there was no wildlife, there was one spot on the horizon line that looked like a bird. When the writer pointed this out, he quickly went over it with his pencil to make it part of the horizon line. The final sentence Nathan constructed read: "I'm waiting on a raft, stuck in the middle of an ocean, stranded, bored, and sinking." This could indicate that he is caught in the middle of a situation that is going on in his life right now, unable to get out of it. He could be bored with it, and can see, whatever it may be, as failing.

Nathan did share that if the raft began to sink in his dream, he would wake up having released semen. The logs drawn creating the raft may even be suggestive of penises; however, this could be overgeneralizing. The fact that Nathan suggested that he would have released semen upon awakening suggests that he may be having nocturnal emissions and/or harbors guilt around past or present nocturnal emissions. The small figure that represented himself on the raft may have been drawn that size in order to show the sensation of the large proportion of the sea and sun in his dream, or it could indicate that he has feelings of insecurity (Oster & Crone, 2004). He may also be withdrawn, depressed, and have feelings of inadequacy (Oster & Crone, 2004). There was no indication of hands, again possibly signaling feelings of inadequacy or even feeling troubled (Oster & Crone, 2004). Although hands were missing, Nathan did include fingers that were long and spike-like that may reveal signs of aggression or hostility (Oster & Crone, 2004).

Recommendations and Conclusions

By comparing all three assessments, overall conclusions can be determined regarding Nathan's characteristics. The fact that Nathan used pencil for all drawings, even when he was able to use coloring media, may conclude that Nathan is afraid to explore any emotions surrounding the drawings he completed since color is known to extract feelings and emotions. In addition, all the drawings, for the most part, lacked symmetry, indicating that Nathan may have inadequate feelings of security in his emotional life (Hammer, 1958). This challenges the score Nathan obtained in the Stimulus Drawing (see Chapter 10) that indicated he may be aware of his emotions and can freely express them through art. All the drawings contained straight-line strokes, which may be present in individuals who tend to be assertive (Hammer, 1958). The drawings of himself in each picture lacked hands, possibly signifying feelings of trouble or inadequacy (Oster & Crone, 2004). In the drawings that contained trees, most of them had two lines for a trunk and a looped crown, possibly displaying impulsive characteristics (Oster & Crone, 2004). All the trees in the pictures either had no or a very minimal root system, which may insinuate that Nathan represses some of his emotions (Oster & Crone, 2004). Each picture was lacking a definite ground line, which could imply that Nathan is vulnerable to stress or that he is unstable (Oster & Crone, 2004). Both the ATDA and SDT (see Chapter 10) uncovered possible unconscious thoughts of escape from some situation in his life.

From reviewing the drawings, the writer concluded that Nathan falls between Lowenfeld and Brittain's (1975) Schematic Stage (7–9 years) and Gang Age (9–12 years). The drawings were more conceptual rather than perceptual. They also had a bold, direct representation with the organization of objects being mostly two-dimensional with there being little overlap; however, there was some awareness to detail. In addition, Nathan expressed the self-consciousness of his drawings. There still seemed to be no understanding of shade and shadow; although, there was less exaggeration of body parts and more stiffness of figures.

The administrant suggests that although there seemed to be no significant indications of problems that were a cause for concern from reviewing these three assessments, she feels that Nathan may still benefit from occasional Art Therapy to release any stress he may be encountering. It may also be beneficial in that it may help him become more in touch with his feelings and emotions, and he may learn ways of expressing them. Art Therapy can also be used as an opportunity to sort out any feelings of trouble or inadequacy that may be occurring, or to explore his impulsivity.

Identified Patient: L

DOB: January 20, 1958

CA: 49

Testing Date: April 1, 2007

Administrant: Barbara Murak

Assessments Administered: ATDA, BATA, PPAT

See Chapters 3 and 9 for further examples regarding L.

Refer to Appendix A for Genogram, Timeline, Behavioral Observations, and Psychosocial Indicators.

The client used the reoccurring black (in the KFD – not included in this book and the PPAT – see Chapter 9) to draw her entire dream. The client drew and filled in her black belt, suggesting sexual preoccupation (Hammer, 1980). The only other color used is brown on the dirty toilet, which could indicate regression to the anal stage (Hammer, 1980). Dirt has a negative connotation, as in admonishing dirty thoughts, clothes or negative feelings (Burns & Kaufman, 1972). Pictures using one color, such as black, seem to occur with some frequency among patients with major depression (Gantt & Tabone, 1998). The use of black in drawing figures, repeated in subsequent assessments, may indicate the client's reoccurring depression (see Chapter 9). Hammer suggests that "black and brown are more common to states of inhibition, repression, and possibly regression" (Hammer, 1980, p. 233). The client commented that she drew bell-bottom pants, and "thinking about them touching the floor would be my worst nightmare," perhaps demonstrating her fear of contamination, both in her dream and in her repeated sexual encounters.

Dream Analysis: "When my bladder is full, I dream I have to use the bathroom. It is always a public facility. But I can't go because either the stalls are occupied or disgustingly dirty, or there is only half a door and people can see me, or there is no door." Final Sentence: "When my bladder is full, I can't go in a public facility when it is disgustingly dirty or people can see me." The client commented afterwards that, "If I resolve my dream, I'm afraid I'll pee myself in real life." The client shows a possible concern with contamination, as was her stated concern regarding dating and having sex with many men.

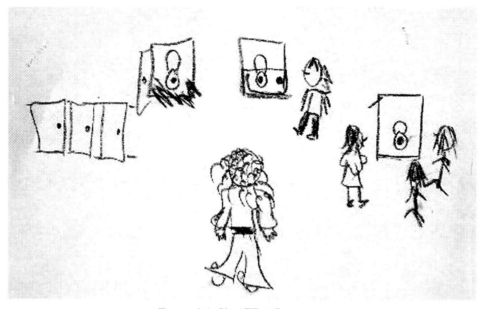

Figure 2.3. L's ATDA Response.

Conclusions

The client's childlike drawings could indicate that in periods of stress, she regresses to the developmental age range preceding that period in her life when she was starved for emotional nourishment from her environment, perhaps preadolescent (Hammer, 1980). Her numerous dating and sexual encounters would indicate that the client is longing to experience nurturing, emotional warmth and interpersonal relationships that were lacking in her childhood. The client seems to be experiencing conflicted feelings of rigidity and lack of control regarding her sexual impulses. This writer would recommend further art therapy to address issues of loneliness, depression, self-esteem, insecurity, and fear of contamination as a result of her promiscuity. All drawings began at the right-hand side of the paper, which may indicate inhibition. Rigidity of her self-drawings indicate keeping herself closed off against the world, while simultaneously keeping her inner impulses under rigid control (Hammer, 1980).

Chapter 3

BELIEF ART THERAPY ASSESSMENT (BATA)

Religiosity and belief have been juxtaposed by science and rational thinking. While they are closely related and certainly interface, they are distinctly different. Moreover, since the seventeenth century Galileo affair, science and religion forged an unwritten contract of nonrelationship. Religious thinkers agreed that the "natural world" was the sole province of the scientists. And scientists agreed to keep their nose out of the "supernatural," or for that matter anything to do with the spiritual. Verily, science circumscribed itself as "value-free."

According to Peck, ". . . there has been a profound separation between religion and science. This divorce . . . more often remarkably amicable – has decreed that the problem of evil should remain in the custody of religious thinkers. With few exceptions, scientists have not even sought visitation rights, if for no other reason than the fact that science is supposed to be value-free." Peck further espoused that for a variety of multifaceted reasons, this separation no longer works. He stated, "There are many compelling reasons for their reintegration – one of them being the problem of evil itself – even to the point of the creation of a science that is no longer value-free" (1983, p. 40).

Today, this partnership has caused scientists and religious thinkers alike to reside as uneasy bedfellows. Yet, it was not always this way. The history of most culture declared an integration of science with the religious and ritualized "spiritual" activities (Dearing, 1983; Dombeck & Karl, 1987; Frank & Frank, 1991; Jung, 1965). By the last century, a profound departure occurred from this plaited marriage. In fact, this duality caused ministerial and health care professions to become formally distinct. The result has ranged from open hostility to mutual cooperation.

Indeed, the religious and spiritual needs have been entrusted to the clergy. Baptism, last rites, confirmation, communion, and even prayer have been relegated to religious leaders. This domain has created a fissure for any clinician who has faced a client's spiritual questions, struggle with faith, and/or desire for forgiveness. There have been several options:

1. Ignoring the spiritual dimension of the patient;
2. Chalking up the patient's thinking as floridly psychotic;
3. Referring the patient to a clergy person without participating in that aspect of care (thus, defeating a systemic approach);
4. Collaborating with a clergy person and working out an interdisciplinary approach to treatment;
5. Or attempting to spiritually counsel the patient.

Dombeck and Karl came up with these additional postulates:

1. Who should assess religious and spiritual needs, and how are these needs assessed by each profession?
2. Would an interdisciplinary approach increase the possibility for spiritual assessment and response to spiritual needs?
3. Is the assessment of spiritual needs important in making correct diagnoses? (1987, p. 184.)

Truly, a holistic approach to a person's wellness includes mind, body, and spirit. And, the premise behind the BATA was to investigate these aforementioned options and questions. Thus, the BATA takes on the assumption that spiritual care is a legitimate part of health care. Even though the clergy and other faith healers have a specified role in this arena, the spiritual needs of a patient require attention and treatment by the entire health care team.

First, however, some definitions are necessary:

Interdisciplinary is defined as a process of combining the myriad talents and skills of professionals necessary to eradicate the problems of a person's condition and contribute to his overall recovery and health.

While related, the terms *religion* and *spiritual* are **not** synonymous:

Religion, an organized system of faith, is defined as an "organized body of thought and experience concerning the fundamental problems of existence."

Spirituality "deals with the life principle that pervades and animates a person's entire being, including emotional and volitional aspects of life . . . The search for meaning and purpose through suffering and the need for forgiveness are elements of the spiritual life" (Dombeck & Karl, 1987, p. 184).

As well, the terms *faith* and *community* require both consideration and definition:

Faith, while often associated with the term "belief," reflects confidence in the trust and value of a person, idea, or thing. Tradition imposed on a belief system gives *rise* to faith. According to the dictionary, faith has also been linked to a belief and trust in God, as well as a religious conviction hinged to a system of religious principles and beliefs. However, one definition that is differentiated from religious dogma unites faith with a belief that does not rest on logical proof or material evidence.

Community demands inclusion since man interfaces with his cultural network and relies on this system for feedback, reinforcement, support, and oftentimes, for parameters within his individualized frame of reference. Ashbrook in his treatise, *be/come Community*, talked about our highway system as being the only true source of communal architecture since it "organizes, channels, connects, and directs our separate yet independent living." In linking community with both a means and way in which to connect with others, he proposed that the means "enables us to break out of the boxes in which we are trapped" (providing an instrument for our intentions), as well as a way to wed us to reality and other people (1971, p. 72–73).

From a systemic perspective, an interdisciplinary and communal approach to treating an identified patient within a family systems framework is not only essential but also fundamental in the treatment of the whole person (see Figure 1.1 in Chapter 1 for elucidation on this concept). Incorporating the spiritual and religious components into treatment requires a tool for assessing whatever nodal events contributed to the disorder and dis-ease of the person. While the Belief Art Therapy Assessment (BATA; fully described in Horovitz, 2002 and at the end of this chapter) offers an instrument for estimation, the reader may not be comfortable with continued exploration of a patient's spiritual belief system. If, in fact, this is the case, then one needs to embrace an interdisciplinary approach and rely on the skills and talents of other professionals within the community

Integrating art therapy with family therapy from an historical perspective requires a systemic orientation. On intake, the administrant needs to join with his patient(s) and construct a three-generation genogram (Guerin & Pendagast, 1976) as detailed in Chapter 1. This historical perspective views the identified patient (I.P.) in context of the family's life cycle and allows the practitioner to review historical events that created the current symptomatolgy within the family's present condition. This enables the therapist to consider the relevancy of the underlying issues as outlined by the critical past events and issues. Moreover, it empowers the clinician with the armament necessary for adequately combating the issues with empathy and direction. With these tools, the clinician moves on to the next stage of assessing and diagnosing the I.P. in order to construct a hypothesis for treatment.

Now there are some art therapists who arguably contend that assessment and diagnosis is unnecessary for treatment. While assessment and diagnosis may not be the axis point for all art therapists, the authors herein suggest that one cannot do adequate treatment without it. Would a doctor prescribe pharmaceutical medication without assessing and determining the causality? Most likely, not. Assessment and diagnosis encompass the full range of the patient from a holistic perspective. Like the good doctor, exploring every avenue when pursuing the etiology of the system, is the hallmark of an able, well-armed clinician. And when wrestling with physical, psychological, and/or emotional disorders and dis-ease, one needs all the accouterments that he or she can muster. (Indeed, "Dis" is an old Roman name for the mythological underworld. When considering how disease enters the body and finds an opening into health where functioning breakdowns, the concept of dis-comfort and dis-function seems quite applicable.)

While a number of assessment tests abound as indicated by this **when indicated**, the Belief Art Therapy Assessment test (BATA) should be deployed when a client questions his or her belief system and/or brings up issues of faith (wavering or not). (However, it should be underscored that one should employ the BATA **only** when warranted. The reason is that when florid, psychotic thinking is present conducting the test in its entirety can in fact exacerbate this condition, plaguing emotionally disturbed individuals.) So the adage is to conduct the BATA *only* when the patient questions or brings up his belief/spiritual dimension on interview or within the aforementioned testing component. Moreover, it is conducted *only* when the information might lead to an improved understanding of the patient as opposed to contributing to further deterioration of his condition. Furthermore, even after the patient reveals his spiritual struggle by way of the BATA, it is wholly possible that he may not be ready to explore his "spiritual dimension" since this involves abstract thinking. If, in fact, the patient's thinking is formal, rigid, and concrete, then the therapist needs to walk this line with trepidation and *always* respect the client's lead.

Conducting these tests offers a vantage point for assessing treatment perspectives. But no matter what the etiology or current condition of the IP, it is always imperative to return to the origins of mourning and loss (Horovitz-Darby, 1991). For the benchmark in exploring mourning and loss sets the table for spiritual recovery and mental health.

In abiding by this, one is reminded of the task beset by the universal Job. The biblical yarn of Job, who in one day lost all of his fortune, husbandry, and ten children, is a remarkable tale of a man who never lost faith in God. Even though he was tested by misfortune and destitution, Job's steadfast belief resulted in God reinstating his lot with additional riches, family, and good fortune. The moral, that through faith all can be restored, is indeed strong medicine.

Next, the reader will find some examples of the BATA.

Identified Patient: L

DOB: January 20, 1958

CA: 49

Testing Date: April 1, 2007

Administrant: Barbara Murak

Assessments Administered: ATDA, BATA, PPAT

See Chapters 2 and 9 for further examples regarding L.

Refer to Appendix A for Genogram, Timeline, Behavioral Observations, and Psychosocial Indicators.

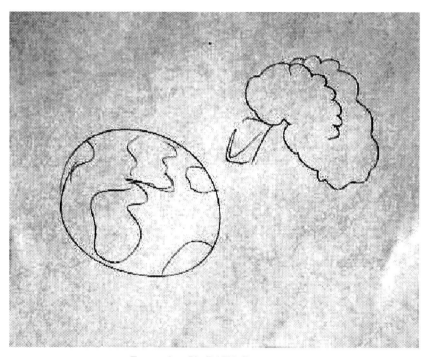

Figure 3.1. L's BATA Response.

The client related learning much from her experiences and spiritual readings, and the subsequent discussion of especially meaningful spiritual books led the writer to administering the BATA. Assessment began following some of the suggested history-taking questions in the *Spiritual Art Therapy: An Alternate Path* (Horovitz, 2002). The client used a pencil and hastily drew a world and a cloud, with an arrow going between them, stating "Our lives are what we THINK about our lives; like Byron Katie's 'Is it true?'" The client explained she was raised Catholic, but that she never wanted to be Catholic, and was "forced" (to be Catholic) until she was 16 years old. The client states now she is "spiritual, but not religious." When this writer asked the second directive, the client said she doesn't believe in the opposite of God or the devil, only that there was good and evil, which is open to interpretation. "I might think someone does something bad, but they do not think of it that way at all. And what can be bad ends up a good thing. Like breaking up with someone bad at the time, but then you meet someone better and in the end it is good. Or falling in love with someone seems good, but then he beats you up and it ends up bad." These statements reflect the client's obvious projection. The use of pencil after using chalk pastels for all other assessments, and the simplicity of drawn image may indicate her tiredness at the end of our two-hour session, but was consistent with her other drawings in the Gang Age 9–12 years, developmental stage (Lowenfeld & Brittain, 1975). Her artwork was so faintly drawn that maybe she lacks conviction of her beliefs. The client is an artist, but her drawing did not exhibit any talent to place her at an adult stage of development. Fowler's Stage 4 would describe the client's current belief system. She transitioned from Catholic to "spiritual," as she puts it, at 45 years of age, which is consistent with Fowler's statement that many adults do not embark on this journey until their late thirties or early forties (Fowler, 1981).

Conclusions

The client's childlike drawings could indicate that in periods of stress, she regresses to the developmental age range preceding that period in her life when she was starved for emotional nourishment from her environment, perhaps preadolescent (Hammer, 1980). Her numerous dating and sexual encounters would indicate that the client is longing to experience nurturing, emotional warmth, and interpersonal relationships that were lacking in her childhood. The client seems to be experiencing conflicted feelings of rigidity and lack of control regarding her sexual impulses. This writer would recommend further art therapy to address issues of loneliness, depression, self-esteem, insecurity, and fear of contamination as a result of her promiscuity. All drawings began at the right-hand side of the paper, which may indicate inhibition. Rigidity of her self-drawings indicate keeping herself closed off against the world, while simultaneously keeping her inner impulses under rigid control (Hammer, 1980).

Identified Patient: Pam

DOB: August 1954

CA: 52

Testing Dates: September 27, 2006; March 21, 2007; March 28, 2007

Administrant: Julie Riley

Assessments Administered: BATA, FSA, SDT

See Chapters 6 and 10 for further examples regarding Pam.

Refer to Appendix A for Genogram, Timeline, Behavioral Observations, and Psychosocial Indicators.

According to Lowenfeld and Brittain (1975), Pam's God response falls within the Preschematic Stage of Development, ages 4–7 years; and the opposite of God would be classified at the Scribble Stage, ages 2–4 years.

Though this assessment is designed to begin with an inquiry of spiritual history, this writer opted to remind Pam of a previous session when she expressed a belief in God and her religious affiliation, Jehovah's Witness. Pam was asked to draw or paint what God meant to her. She responded, "I don't think I can do that." So this writer rephrased, "Can you draw or paint how God makes you feel?" Pam responded, "Ok, I can do that." She chose paint and initially exhibited interest in this directive. She began with a smile and appeared to be deriving pleasure from the painting. She talked while she painted the "earth" and a "growing, big tree" reciting, "God is everywhere and part of everything. I don't know how else it could be." After the trunk of her first tree became larger than she wanted, she began showing signs of discomfort. The abandoned attempt of the first tree seemed to reflect disintegration. Similarly, during a study of the Diagnostic Drawing Series, researchers noticed disintegration in tree drawings in 47 percent of head-injured patients compared to 7 percent of the control group during a study gathering information comparing clinical diagnoses and characteristics of art production (Cheyne-King, 1990). Pam continued by adding the smaller tree. She initiated use of the blue paint, allowing a single drop to fall on the paper but became too distracted and frustrated to paint any more. Pam's God response went untitled because upon completion the frustration level was too heightened to discuss the image. Historically, trees have symbolized life and God; "the tree was worshipped among early peoples as a sacred object inhabited by a god" (Hall, 1979, p. 307). Pam's painting might reflect the role God played in her life following the accident (see Appendix A). The trunk-only tree may symbolize her life prior to the accident leaving the second tree to symbolize her rebirth as a different person following the accident. The second tree is more complete; it has a trunk (though unsubstantial when compared with its crown) and branches; the majority of her life has been lived by the "second" person. According to a Jungian paradigm, trees reflect growth, life, and the individual; and more universally, "the tree of life . . . a symbol of the universe and of cosmic renewal – represents both the cyclic transformation of life and the continuity of life, or eternal life" (Kast, 1992, p. 115).

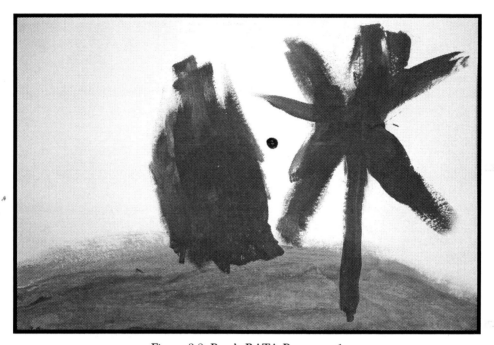

Figure 3.2. Pam's BATA Response 1.

For the directive, "paint the opposite of how God makes you feel," Pam responded using only blue paint and continuous brush stroking. She appeared out of breath while completing this painting, which took approximately 30 minutes of a 60-minute session to complete. Her affect was low and depressed upon completion; and her posture seemed to reflect dejection. Pam entitled her painting *Blue Mess*, which this writer considered an act and product of sublimation. As explained by Kramer, "Sublimation entails establishing a symbolic linkage between some primitive need and another more complex cluster of ideas and actions" (Kramer, 2001, p. 29). The complexity of the subject (God and belief), Pam's product, her physiological response, and her emotional release indicate regressive channeling of inner conflicts and anxieties in combination with a release through creative production.

Kramer's idea of sublimation also postulates "that man's subjective experiences can be linked to the physiological process of tension reduction; that actions which are linked only by a long chain of modification to the gratifications of basic urges can have the power to generate emotions of pleasure and pain" (Kramer, 2001, p. 29). The feelings Pam associated with *Blue Mess* were loneliness and sadness. She verbalized conflict between her housemates and missing the companionship of her sisters. Her "Opposite of God" visual response and verbal association denote isolation and depression. *Blue Mess* is the most expressive painting Pam has done in a session to date with this writer. It provoked dialogue regarding her emotional state oriented in the present as opposed to memories of the past, which was rare. Withrow writes, "The right brain, which communicates in images, is symbolic and emotional, and can tell us what we actually feel" (2004, p. 34). It is often difficult for Pam to communicate her feelings to this writer; and the art from this session motivated a progression in Pam's emotional development.

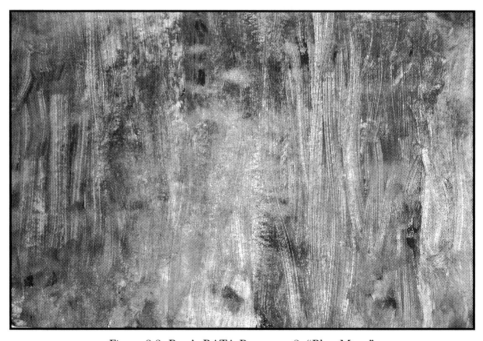

Figure 3.3. Pam's BATA Response 2, "Blue Mess."

Identified Patient: Karla

DOB: September 11, 1985

CA: 22

Testing Date: September 24, 2007

Administrant: Luke M. Sworts

Assessment Administered: BATA

Refer to Appendix A for Genogram, Timeline, Behavioral Observations, and Psychosocial Indicators.

First Directive

When asked to draw what God means to her, Karla took approximately five minutes to create the artwork seen in Figure 3.4. (For color version, see Plate 2, p. 109.) This illustration has a sketchy line quality and has symmetry down its central vertical axis. Two sets of blue clouds with yellow rays emerging are contained in the upper portion of the artwork. The lower hemisphere has a ground line of sorts, shaded in green. At the center, four circles or

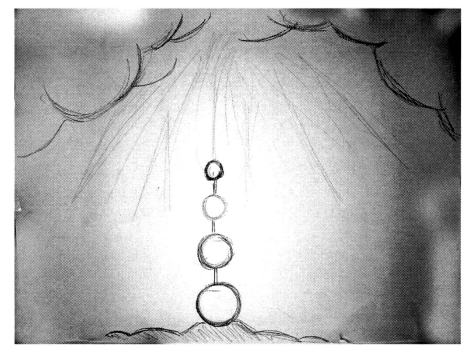

Figure 3.4. Karla's BATA Response 1, "What God means to me."
(For color version, see Plate 2, p. 109.)

spheres, each of different color (red, orange, blue, and purple) and size (largest to smallest), are stacked vertically. Each sphere is connected to its adjacent sphere by a double green line.

Karla explained the illustration as a time when the sunshine pierces through the clouds in a very dramatic fashion and the individual rays are very lucid. She also alluded to that fact that she only thinks of God when "bad things happen" and recalled the suicide of a friend's father. Karla then affirmed that God is a belief-in-self that exists during the course of your life. This interviewer inquired about the nature of the spherical forms and Karla described them as self formation or development over time. Another potential interpretation is that the spheres are representative of Karla's siblings. When asked, Karla revealed she had never seen God as she had drawn and also that she felt "awkward, I dunno . . . I feel I should know, but I don't . . . being asked to represent . . . it's weird, confusing. . . ." Although the client was able to produce a product that covered the entire page, the fact that much of the drawing consisted of empty space may identify her uncertainty regarding the task at hand.

Second Directive

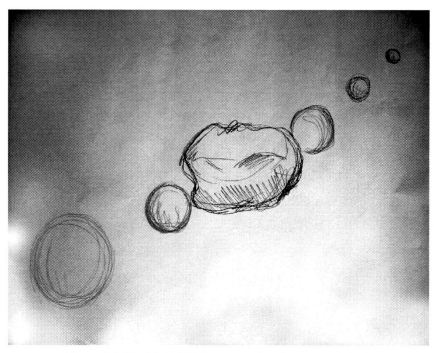

Figure 3.5. Karla's BATA Response 2 – Opposite of God.
(For color version, see Plate 3, p. 110.)

Asked to draw the opposite of God, Karla took approximately three minutes to create the artwork in Figure 3.5. (For color version, see Plate 3, p. 110.) As in the first directive we see the multisized spheres of different colors. However, in this illustration the spheres are aligned along a diagonal axis rising upward from left to right. Furthermore, there is no longer a double line connecting the spheres, but a large brown and black object, identified as a rock or obstacle, placed in the center of the page between two of the spheres. In comparison to the first directive there is an additional sphere, and these five spheres do not appear aligned by size as efficiently as in the first directive. The overall impression of the artwork gives the sense that the objects are floating in space as there is no ground or skyline. The lack of groundline may also be associated with insecurity (Hammer, 1958) in particular, when confronted about her lack of belief system.

Upon inquiry Karla again fumbled for words to describe her illustration, describing the opposite of God as "the thing that holds you back," then again doubting herself and suggesting it was "the impossible." She then recanted, mentioning that obstacles can be good things and thus, she did not think that this was it (the opposite of God). Again, Karla had not seen the opposite of God as she had drawn it. When asked about her feeling state, Karla replied, "pretty good" and added that her drawing was representative of life challenges or difficulty. This interviewer sensed a relief in the client upon completion of the task and suspects her emotional state is more reflective of the task being finished, rather than her contentment with the finished product and her associated understanding of it.

Discussion

This administration of the BATA should be viewed with limited clinical implications. Although administered according to the guidelines as outlined in Horovitz's Spiritual Art Therapy (2002), a therapeutic relationship had not been established. Moreover, the client had not demonstrated a questioning of faith or spiritual concerns, both of which are indicators to administer the BATA. Lastly, the interviewer (and author of this paper) has limited training and experience in interpreting the results of the BATA. Accordingly, the results of this test should not be considered clinically significantly.

Interpreting the results of the BATA can be done quantitatively as well as qualitatively (Horovitz, 2002). Not only will we look at the objective nature of the drawing itself (composition, line quality, color) our discussion will also focus on the quality of the experience. Thus, we will examine the client's verbal and nonverbal responses in relation to the artwork produced to gain insight into the client's holistic belief system.

Considering the size of both drawings, we neither see a diminished drawing nor an expansive drawing. In both instances the subject matter fits on the page and to a certain degree covers the entire page. Hammer (1958) hypothesizes that both extremes are related to feelings of realistic self-esteem. Accordingly, the size of the artwork does not reveal any insight into an over or underinflated ego on the part of the client, but suggests that the client is comfortable within her environment. Meanwhile, the indecisive and light nature of the strokes may indicate some discomfort with the subject nature. Hammer (1958) postulated that indecisive or sketchy lines may be emphasized when a client experiences anxiety or hesitancy. Given the client's verbal responses to the directives one can assume she was not certain in the description of her spiritual belief systems.

In regards to the symmetry we see in directive one, Hammer (1958) notes that strict symmetry is associated with obsessive-compulsive tendencies. However, the artwork produced by this client does not demonstrate such rigid symmetry that a diagnosis should be further examined. More likely, this tendency is reflective of certain personality characteristics inherent in the individual. Lastly, a quick note on color; although color may bear significant emotional importance (Hammer, 1958), the lack of predominant color, or areas of overemphasized color, prevents a formal hypothesis as to its importance within this artwork. Additional inquiries to the client regarding her interpretation of the use of color may bear fruitful results.

Examining the comments associated with the artwork produced allows us to identify the belief system stage of the client. Identifying herself as a Catholic, yet having no practices, rituals, or significant religious experiences suggests the client has, at best, low to moderate spiritual identity. One must assume her identity as a Catholic is based on familial roots. Had the interviewer collected additional information on the three-generation genogram, one would likely see patterns of religious practice associated with the Catholic faith. Such characteristics as described above are suggestive of Stage 3: Synthetic-Conventional Faith (Fowler, 1981).

However, the client comments that she gets strength from family *and* friends, as well as her own self-confidence. Accordingly, we must recognize her growth beyond family. Such development is characteristic of adolescents and young adults, as Stage 3 indicates (Fowler, 1981). Fowler (1981) calls Stage 3 "principally a *tacit* system" or unexamined system. Clearly, the uncertainty on part of the client in defining her artwork or explaining her relationship with God supports this concept.

In closing, Stage 3: Synthetic-Conventional Faith can be a stagnant place for adults. If situations or contexts do not provoke the need for further examination or self-exploration, an individual's system of faith will not develop (Fowler, 1981). The task of the BATA itself may have sparked an internal examination within the client. Similarly, if left alone, Stage 3 may also break down to lower concepts of faith systems.

BATA Format and Directives

History Taking

Name, Age, Religion, and Career (if applicable)

<u>Questions:</u>

1. What is you religious affiliation?
2. Have there ever been any changes in your religious affiliation?
3. When did these changes take place (if applicable) and what were the circumstances that caused this change?
4. What is the level of your present involvement with your church, temple, or faith community?
5. What is your relationship with your pastor, rabbi, priest, or spiritual leader?
6. Do you have any religious practices that you find particularly meaningful?
7. What kind of relationship do you have with God if applicable?
8. What gives you special strength and meaning?
9. Is God involved in your problems? (Depending on how this is answered, you might want to clarify whether or not the subject involves God in his problems and/or blames God for his problems.)
10. Have you ever had a feeling of forgiveness from God?

N.B. All of these questions need not be asked and also depending on personality and psychological parameters, one may choose to skip this section altogether since it may exacerbate psychosis.

First Directive

   Please remember that the manner in which a subject is presented with the request to delineate his belief system is all-important. The administrat could begin the topic by stating something like, "Have you ever thought about how the universe was created and who or what was responsible for its creation?" Then once a dialogue regarding the topic is started, the interviewer could actually lead into the art task itself by stating, "Many people have a belief in God; if you also have a belief in God, would you draw, paint, or sculpt what God **means** to you." The instruction should be stated exactly as it is written since any deviation from the original intent might imply subject bias. The reason for the words **"means to you"** is essential. Direct representation may be offensive in some religious/cultural background.

If a prospective subject is an atheist or agnostic, the administrant might simply request that the subject attempt to delineate what it is he or she believes in. If the subject believes in nothing, one could ask the subject to define that in the media.

However, if the subject defines himself/herself as an agnostic/atheist, some questions might be:

1. Have you ever believed in God?
   If the answer is yes, one might then ask:
2. What caused you to no longer believe in God and when did that occur?

(One could still ask questions 5, 8, and 10 as stated above)

Second Directive

Some people create the opposite of God simultaneously with the above directive of creating what God means to them. If, however, the subject does not, then state, "Some people believe that there is an opposite of God. If you believe there is an opposite force, could you also draw, paint, or sculpt that?"

Naturally, the same post assessment interrogation can proceed following the latter request.

The BATA can be scored cognitively according to Lowenfeld and Brittain (1975) using the same parameters that are outlined in the CATA assessment (Horovitz, 1988, 1999).

Post-Assessment Interrogation

1. Could you explain what you have made and what that means to you?
2. Have you ever witnessed or seen God as you have delineated your artwork?
3. How do you feel about what you have just made?

Moreover, let the subject talk freely about his or her artwork and record significant verbal associates to the work produced.

Chapter 4

BENDER-GESTALT II

The Bender-Gestalt was first introduced by Lauretta Bender in 1938 through her innovative monograph, *A Visual Motor Gestalt and Its Clinical Use*. Her premise was that the function of an integrated organism responds to a "given constellation of stimuli as a whole." She further proposed that the "integrative processes of the nervous system occur(ed) in constellations, patterns, and gestalten . . . and that the organism determine(d) the pattern of the response" (p. 3–4).

Indeed, the original Bender-Gestalt test was able to identify mental retardation, disabilities (such as reading), organic brain abnormalities, personality dynamics, psychotic dysfunctioning, cultural differences, and so forth. According to Piotrowksi (1995), "the Bender-Gestalt continues to be ranked among the ten top instruments in use . . . evident across all age groups" (p. 1272). While the original test only employed nine designs, because of developmental advances based on age and abilities, the test was re-designed with card designs to copy for 8 and under and over 8 by disallowing certain designs as they became progressively more difficult to replicate. To optimize the test, children below the age of 8 would be administered the new, easier items as well as the original items on the 1938 Bender-Gestalt test modeled by Bender. Ages 4 year to 7 years 11 months would be given cards 1–12 and anyone 8 years and older would start with card number 5 and end at card number 16. Thus a process for new item calibration was employed using a model that independently estimated item difficulty and subject ability. The new calibration system involved a procedure that systematically ranked original and new test cards along a continuum of difficulty (Rasch, 1960). (N.B.: difficulty, being defined as how hard it might be for a person to copy the design relative to the existing Bender-Gestalt.)

A Recall Test was also introduced that requires that the examinee illustrate the designs from memory (immediately following the test). Although the recall test has no limits, the recorder ascertains how long it takes to complete each section.

The Global Scoring system was employed to assist in evaluating the over-all quality of the reproduced designs (both Copy and Recall sections of the test). Moreover, the Global Scoring system evaluated the overall qualitative aspects of the results with a 5-point rating system (from 0–4) consisting of the following criteria:

Scoring for the Global Scoring System is as follows (Brannigan & Decker, 2003, p. 20):

0 = no resemblance, random drawing, scribbling, lack of design
1 = Slight – vague resemblance
2 = Some – moderate resemblance
3 = Strong – close resemblance, accurate reproduction
4 = Nearly perfect

Individual scores for each item (using this Global Scoring System, adapt-ed from the earlier Qualitative Scoring System) could yield a total score of 0–52 for examinees below age 8 and 0–48 for subjects 8 and older.

Of importance was a new observation form that allowed the administrant to record and document pertinent information for interpretation and report writing. In addition, to the new calibrated designs two new supplemental tests, the Motor Test and the Perception Test were established along with a new Global Scoring System. (These supplemental tests were designed to dis-tinguish motor and/or perceptual tests that would negatively affect the sub-ject's performance and are completed after the Copy and Recall tests are completed.)

Scoring for the Motor Test is as follows (Brannigan & Decker, 2003, p. 21):

1 = Line touches both end point and does not leave the box. Line may touch the border but cannot go over it.
0 = Line extends outside the box or does not touch both end points.

A total of twelve (12) points is possible.

Scoring for the Perceptual Test is as follows (Brannigan & Decker, 2003, p. 21):

Each correct response is scored one (1) point. Each incorrect response is scored zero (0) points. A total of ten (10) points is possible.

For more comprehensive information on the test and its administration, the reader is referred to the examiner's manual of the Bender© Visual Motor Gestalt Test, Second Edition by Brannigan and Decker (2003).

Below are some samples of the Bender-Gestalt II to offer the reader some insight in its properties and use for assessment, diagnosis, and treatment.

Identified Patient: M.S.

DOB: January 22, 1955

CA: 52

Administrant: Jaime Balduf

Testing Dates: January-April 2007

Assessment Administered: Bender-Gestalt II

Refer to Appendix A for Genogram, Timeline, Behavioral Observations, and Psychosocial Indicators.

M.S. was very cooperative with the art therapist when asked to complete the Bender Visual-Motor Gestalt Test. He began immediately after the directions were given. M.S. exhibited no signs of physical impediments while taking the test, despite his history of brain injury and eye surgery. While working, M.S. seemed to be excessively concerned with the details of each design. He erased a few times, yet was unsuccessful at correcting his errors. During the copy phase, M.S. constantly looked back and forth between each design and his own drawings. M.S. took each horizontal design and drew them vertically, rotating the left to right sequence of drawing into a top to bottom

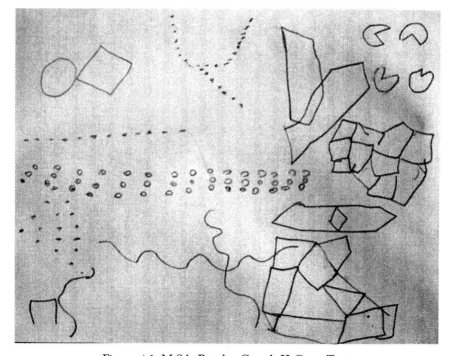

Figure 4.1. M.S.'s Bender-Gestalt II Copy Test.

sequence. According to Brannigan and Decker, this distortion of the gestalt and severe rotation of images is common with brain injury (2003).

M.S. became increasingly frustrated when attempting to copy the three-dimensional designs of numbers 14 and 16. As in his house drawing (not included in this book), he flattened the various sides of the image. M.S. took 11 minutes and 32 seconds to complete this section. According to these results of the copy section M.S. falls within the average class, with scores of 29, 93, 32.04, and 45 (Brannigan & Decker, 2003). When asked to recall the previous images, M.S. attempted to redraw three of the images and then tried to reconstruct the three-dimensional designs. However, as he became more agitated with his inability to redraw these images, M.S. began to replace the square shapes with circles until he said "I can't." The recall test marked his moderate perseveration on the circle shapes of design numbers one and two and indicated the cognitive affects of his brain injury (Brannigan & Decker, 2003). This portion lasted five minutes and 50 seconds. His scores in this section were extremely low − 5, 40, 0.00, and 10. For both the motor and perception sections of the Bender-Gestalt II, M.S. placed in the 76–100 percentile range, receiving raw scores of 12 and 10 (Brannigan & Decker, 2003).

The results of M.S.'s Bender-Gestalt II test indicate the implications of his brain injury through his rotation and distortion of designs. Despite these difficulties, his motor and perception skills have remained in tact.

Conclusion and Summation

Various aspects found throughout the artwork of M.S. reveal high levels of emotional repression, feelings of covert aggression, and possible insecurities surrounding his family and social abilities. These factors, as well as his preoccupation with the past, may therefore be intensifying M.S.'s levels of anxiety and stress. In order to relieve these feelings, it is important for M.S. to gain a sense of security and to improve his social skills through group participation. Because M.S. has responded well to working with art materials and can express his ideas through imagery, further art therapy sessions are highly recommended. Art therapy could aid M.S. in identifying factors that may be causing his anxiety, help him to develop coping skills and cues, and give him further opportunity to explore and identify his emotions. At the least, M.S. would greatly benefit from having art as a mode of expression and release.

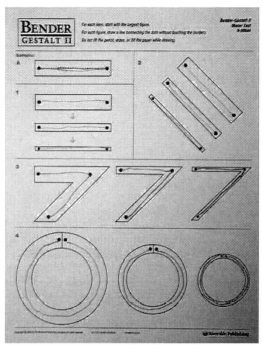

Figure 4.2. M.S.'s Bender-Gestalt II Motor Response.

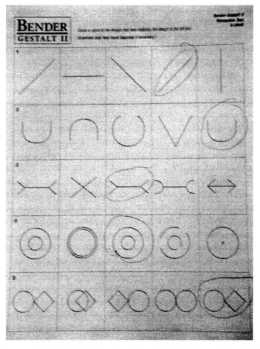

Figure 4.3. M.S.'s Bender-Gestalt II Perception Test.

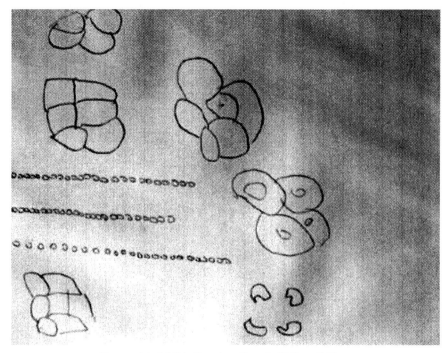

Figure 4.4. M.S.'s Bender-Gestalt II Recall Test.

Client: B

CA: 23

DOB: July 16, 1983

Testing Date: October 13, 2006; October 14, 2006; November 21, 2006

Administrant: Jenn DeRoller

Test Administered: Bender-Gestalt II

Refer to Appendix A for Genogram, Timeline, Behavioral Observations, and Psychosocial Indicators.

B eagerly began the assessment, revealing an increase in frustration throughout testing. Physical observations affecting the assessment are related to her dextral orientation and evidence of an abnormal hand grip. Throughout the testing B appeared to become more frustrated, erased frequently and was seemly consumed with detail. She scored a total of 46 in the copy test, and was placed in the 97.72 percentile (Brannigan & Decker, 2003).

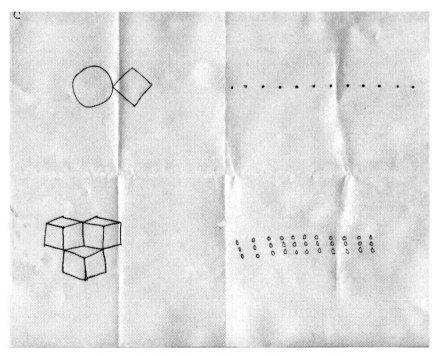

Figure 4.5. B's Bender-Gestalt II Copy Test 1.

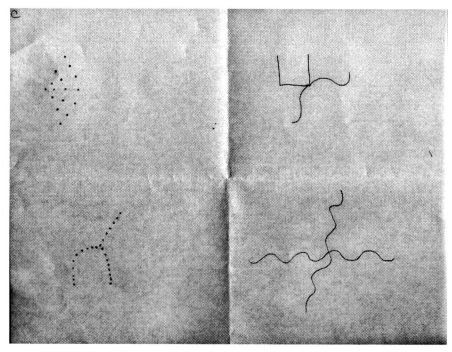

Figure 4.6. B's Bender-Gestalt II Copy Test 2.

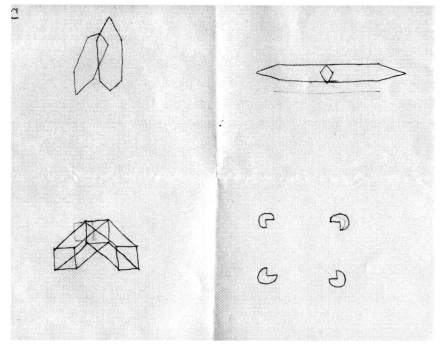

Figure 4.7. B's Bender-Gestalt II Copy Test 3.

In the recall section B appeared to be more frustrated and could only remember seven of the 12 designs. B began creating her own images as a way to compensate for her inability to remember. Her total score was 26 and she was ranked in 85.69 percentile (Brannigan & Decker, 2003).

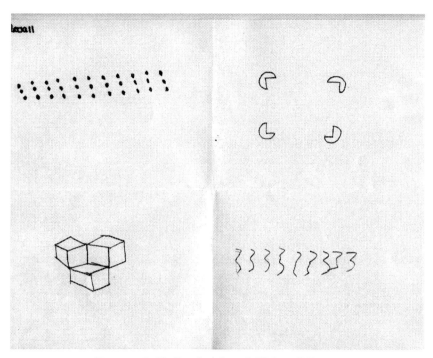

Figure 4.8. B's Bender-Gestalt II Recall Test 1.

During the motor test B appeared to have some difficulty manipulating the pencil inside the lines. She claimed this task was difficult because she was left-handed. Her total score was 12 and she ranked in the 51–100th percentile (Brannigan & Decker, 2003). B spent a total of 15 seconds to complete the perception test. Her total score was 10 and she ranked in the 51–100th percentile (Brannigan & Decker, 2003).

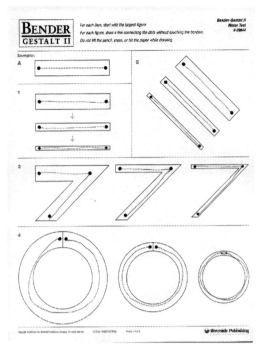

Figure 4.9. B's Bender-Gestalt II Motor Response.

Conclusion and summation

Although B revealed some anxiety and frustration in the completion of the test she scored high in the percentile rank, classifying her in higher-than-average levels. She revealed a great deal of frustration in the recall phase and began to draw designs she indicated she "thought" she remembered, but were not in the test. She also indicated her frustration when she was not allowed to lift her pencil or erase during the motor test.

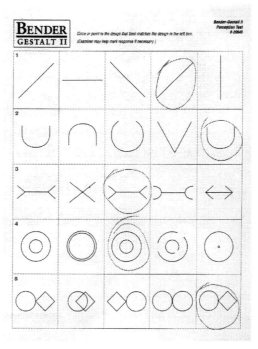

Figure 4.10. B's Bender-Gestalt II Perception Test Response 1.

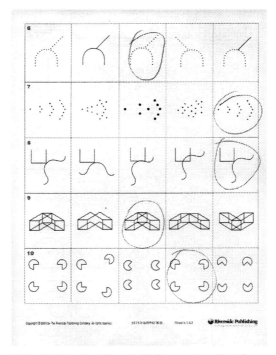

Figure 4.11. B's Bender-Gestalt II Perception Test Response 2.

Chapter 5

COGNITIVE ART THERAPY
ASSESSMENT (CATA)

In the late 1980s, Horovitz published her first rendition of the Cognitive Art Therapy Assessment (CATA). This assessment tool's beauty is that it is guised as an open-ended studio activity and thus little to no stress is involved on the subject's part. Since it does not feel like a "test" because the directive is open-ended (as will be viewed by the instructional below), the client is virtually unaware that his or her response can later be measured for cognitive and developmental change on pretest/posttest measure when utilizing Lowenfeld and Brittain's (1975) developmental scoring system (based on norms for Art Education) or using Horovitz's Adult, Artistic or Brain Injured Stages and scoring system (Horovitz, 2002). Indeed, these artistic developmental stages offer a "snapshot" for the art therapist when beginning treatment planning and preparing to use two and three-dimensional media to facilitate emotional, physical, cognitive, and spiritual recovery.

The following directional is taken from this source below:

Horovitz-Darby, E. G. (1988). Art therapy assessment of a minimally language skilled deaf child. Proceedings from the 1988 University of California's Center on Deafness Conference: *Mental Health Assessment of Deaf Clients: Special Conditions.* Little Rock, Arkansas: ADARA.

COGNITIVE ART THERAPY ASSESSMENT

This procedure has been developed to complement rather than duplicate the multidisciplinary teams' clinical findings. It concentrates on methods whereby art therapy can prove the participant's personality in a unique manner.

It offers open-ended creative activities with pencil, paint, and clay. The dual appeal both towards regression and towards progress to formed expression inherent in all art activities is utilized. In addition, the three media's propensity to elicit specific kinds of behavior is an essential source of information.

- Typically, <u>line drawing</u> elicits intellectually controlled expression as well as storytelling that may be factual or dominated by fantasy.
- <u>Paint</u> raises the emotional key and invites the expression of affect and moods. This might lead to a loosening of controls and/or to flooring of the ego with raw affect.
- <u>Clay</u> invites regression to playful behavior that easily takes on oral, anal, phallic, or genital character. Clay also readily elicits sustained efforts at constructive integration, even in severely disorganized people.

SET-UP

The procedure should be planned to last at least a full hour, one and half-hours are preferable. The session is on the whole conducted as a model art therapy session. Art materials should be set up in advance. This should include:

1. Soft pencil, eraser and white 8" x 11" bond paper.
2. Complete set of poster paint not including orange and violet and also omitting green and brown – set out in an ice cube tray or similar container that allows mixing paints. Two yellows and both ultramarine and turquoise shades of blue for mixing green. Two compartments filled with white to allow mixing lighter colors. An additional empty tray for mixing additional colors. 18" x 24" paper.
3. Ceramic clay, simple clay tools (they can be improvised – sharpened pencils, tongue depressors, etc.), container for mixing clay slip, container for water, hand lotion, paraphernalia for protecting participants and environment must not be forgotten (aprons, newspaper, sponges, etc.)

PROCEDURE

You have a choice to Draw, Paint, and make whatever you want from Clay. You can do all three.

With which (medium) would you like to start?

As the subject chooses his art materials, the art therapist will ask whether, where, and how he has previously used the materials. The art therapist does not interfere while the subject draws. Later on, the art therapist may offer comment, suggestions, advice, or active help when appropriate.

THINGS FOR THE ART THERAPIST TO THINK ABOUT WHEN WRITING UP THE RESULTS: FOCUS OF OBSERVATION

1. <u>Drawing</u>: (a) Developmental stage; (b) motor coordination; (c) Perceptual problems; (d) Reality perception; (e) Thought disorder; (f) Family dynamics
2. <u>Color</u>: effect, mood, e.g., response to the excitement of color (anxious, eager, able):
   * to handle the excitement of color, overwhelmed; color preference; response
   * to the miracle of mixing green; emotional response; can the client use the newly mixed colors? Does he/she understand the principle implied in mixing colors?
3. <u>Clay</u>: capacity for integration; propensity for specific kinds of regression (undifferentiated, playful, oral, anal, aggressive, phalli, etc.) capacity to reintegrate after initial regression.

QUALITY OF THE ARTWORK

1. No product:
   Withdrawal
   Playful experimentation, play
   Destructive behavior
2. Product in the service of defense:
   Banal common stereotype
   Personal stereotype
   Bizarre stereotype
   Doing and undoing
3. Product in the service of primitive discharge:
   Chaotic
   Aggressive
   Obliterating
4. Attempt at formed expression:
   Successful (a product with evocative power, inner consistency)
   Nearly successful
   Failed (when and how did it fail?)
5. Comparison of the art work in the three media offered:
   Similarity
   Dissimilarity
   Incongruence

Is there any material that stimulates extraordinary process or regression?

FORMAL QUALITIES OF ART WORK

- Empty, full; dull, original; fragmented, integrated; static, in motion; rigid, fluid; frantic; bizarre, etc.
- Color over form; form over color
- Skill, talent

SUBJECT MATTER

What themes emerge? Note whether there is any contradiction between overtly stated subject matter and the message conveyed by the work itself.

THE CLIENT'S ATTITUDES

1. General:
   Cooperative, withdrawn, rebellious, suspicious, ambivalent, clinging, integrating, charming, distractible, anxious, intensity, etc. (changes?)
2. Towards his work:
   Highly invested, indifferent, proud, denigrating, self-destructive
3. Towards the art materials:
   Preferences, dislikes
4. Towards suggestions and/or help:
   Oblivious, negative, oh yes! (understanding)
   Dependent but able to integrate help, dependent (bottomless pit of needfulness)

- DID ANY LEARNING TAKE PLACE?
- ANY INDICATION OR CAPACITY TO MASTER INNER RESOURCES IN ART?
- DO OBSERVATIONS CONCUR WITH OR CONTRADICT TEAM'S FINDINGS?
- DID ART ACTIVITY CONTRIBUTE TO EXPRESSION OF MATERIAL NOT OTHERWISE ACCESSIBLE?
- COULD ART ACTIVITIES CONTRIBUTE TO EGO STRENGTH?

GUIDELINES FOR EVALUATION PROCEDURES: FOCUS OF OBSERVATION IN EACH OF THE 3 MEDIA

1. The chronological age must always be taken into consideration when evaluating developmental stage.
2. Both art process and art product should be observed.

3. Observations of art work in one medium will sometimes complement or contradict findings in another medium. Note unevenness of performance, sequence of work done.

I. <u>DRAWING</u>

   A. <u>Developmental stage of drawings:</u>
     1. Scribble
     2. Capacity to produce controlled configurations – circle, triangle, square, etc.
     3. Early representation of the human figure: (predominance of head and limbs. Omission of trunk)
     4. Later representation – trunk appears; limbs form trunk, whole people
     5. Spatial representation: no directness; baseline; fold-over; overlapping; attempts at visual perspective

   B. <u>Signs of constitutional problems:</u>
   These signs can be seen more clearly in drawing than in work with the other materials; however, they should be noted wherever they appear.
     1. Eye-hand coordination?
     2. Problems with fine motor control? Ability to control pencil.
     3. Form perception – ability to produce the basic forms (circle, square, cross, triangle, letters, numbers)
     4. Left – right dominance established?
     5. Reversals or confused directions?
     6. Space discrimination – foreground/background difficulty?
     7. Ease of awkwardness in handling the art material

   C. <u>Facets of personality:</u>
     1. Use of total space, placement of people and objects; directness (framing?, objects afloat?, objects unrelated?)
     2. Size of elements and their relations to each other (this must be considered in relationship to chronological age of participant)
     3. Body image intact; omissions; fragmentations; distortions; bizarre elements. Faces, facial features complete, omissions, distortions; bizarre element; expressions.
     4. Drawing stroke-pressure, broken lines, tentative quality, modulation, continuity, etc. This must be considered in relation to the subject's chronological age.
     5. Omissions, shadings, erasures, transparencies, overemphasis? When corrections are made note whether there is improvement; repetition of the same mistake: deterioration?
     6. Emotional content – joyful, free, pressured, aggressive, boxed-in, etc.
     7. Personal expression or stereotype?

II. PAINTING

A. Developmental stage of painting:

1. Kinesthetic pleasure - squiggle – selection of specific color not important
2. Single areas of massive color; color blobs
3. Separation into different areas of color
4. Color and line combine in representational work and in designs Color modulation through mixing and sensitivity to color relationships. Intellectual comprehension of the principle of mixing color.

B. Facets of personality:

Reaction to paint; strongly attracted to color; able to handle it; reluctant to use it; overwhelmed by it?

- Does color dominate form, swallow, or drown it?
- Is color subordinate to form and subject matter?

C. Specific color preferences and their possible symbolic meeting:

- Hot or cool colors predominate? Dark colors, pastel colors, muddy colors?
- Is there a balance between hot and cool colors?
- Where are emotionally loaded colors placed? (in sky, ground, middle area)
- Overlay, painting one color over another (hiding?)
- Free intermingling of colors or separation of colors?
- Indiscriminate mixing – desire to smear, loss of control, mud?
- Exploration of combinations of color?
- Sequence of color use
- Response to the miracle of green, brown, and other mixed colors
- Ability to use colors that are mixed
- Does mood change with color change?
- Brush stroke, pressure, broken lines, scattered, movement, predominance of vertical and horizontal or curved line
- Personal expression or stereotype?
- Paint as a way of access to fantasy life?

III. CLAY

A. Developmental stage of clay modeling:

1. Clay used playfully; what kind of play?
2. Clay – patted down flat – flat representational work; gingerbread people
3. Clay – squeezed, punched; small differentiated shapes stuck together

4. Use of whole hand – ball, upright forms reminiscent of block building
5. Sculptural form attained: figures assembled from their various parts; simply stuck together; well-joined to make a whole. The sculpture is conceived as a whole from the beginning.
6. Face: features incised in clay; stuck onto the clay; conceived as structure. Note particularly nose (hole, stuck-on protrusion, protruding element of face).

B. Facets of Personality:
1. Enjoying the "feel" of clay? Afraid, repelled by it? Open to experimentation?
2. Capacity for integration? Specific kinds of regression (undifferentiated, playful, oral, anal).
3. Ability to regress and finally re-integrate? Immediately re-integrate?
4. Ability to learn and later recall (after some brief instruction) how to work with clay.
5. Structural elements – faulty connection between parts? Holes, tunnels, hiding place, lack of stability, balance, noting upright, relationship of parts to each other?
6. Emotional content of clay work – playful, imagination, fantasy, bizarre qualities, rigidity, stereotype, aggressive, jabbing?
7. If clay is painted-realistic, symbolic color, bizarre colors?

GENERAL ASSESSMENT AS SEEN THROUGH ART ACTIVITY

1. Outstanding developmental capacities, deficits, deviations, visual-motor functioning. Developmental stage as seen in artwork. If deficits is it possible that they are constitutional and/or emotional, cultural?
2. Self-image: sexual identity, self-esteem, ego ideals.
3. Perception of self in relation to others. Individuation, strong emotional attachments symbiosis?
4. Sense of reality. Distortions of self and body parts, depersonalization?
5. Though processes, ability to conceptualize, memory, judgment, concrete or abstract thinking?
6. Defenses – and dangers defended against.
7. Capacity for other gratifications – not art but playful manipulation of materials.
8. Potential to learn, to master, to function on a higher level, environmental, or cultural factors that might be influential.

9. Temperamental assessment as seen in art session, mood quality – exuberant, hesitant, overwhelmed by anxiety, etc. Activity level – hyperactive, deliberate, reflective, attention span approach or withdrawal? Adaptability or construction.

10. Capacity for ego gratification through art. Capacity for ego maturation through art.

Additionally, when considering the scoring mechanism for the CATA subsections of drawing, painting and clay, the reader should refer to Appendix B, which outlines the stages according to Lowenfeld and Brittain (1975), Horovitz (2002), and others.

Here are samples of the CATA with various populations and clients.

Identified Patient: S

DOB: 2000

CA: 6 years old

Testing Dates: February 26, 2006; March 6, 2006; March 27, 2006

Administrant: Jacob Atkinson

Assessments Administered: CATA, PPAT, SDT

See Chapters 1, 9, and 10 for further examples regarding S.

Refer to Appendix A for Genogram, Timeline, Behavioral Observations, and Psychosocial Indicators.

> *Paint Response:* Schematic Stage, 7–9 year-old, Lowenfeld & Brittain
> *Clay Response:* Preschematic Stage, 4–7 year-old, Lowenfeld & Brittain
> *Pencil Response:* Schematic Stage, 7–9 year-old, Lowenfeld & Brittain
> *Overall Response:* Schematic Stage, 7–9 year-old, Lowenfeld & Brittain

Paint Response

S chose to paint first. When asked if she knew how to mix colors, she stated that she knew how and did not need a demonstration. She began by painting the groundline, followed next by outlining and filling in the giraffe. She finished by painting the flower. S was quick to solve problems encountered during the painting portion of the CATA, such as requesting black paint for the giraffe's tail, which was not given at the beginning of the assessment. S explained the entire process of what she was doing while she worked. According to Hammer (1980), a long neck may imply difficulty controlling and directing instinctual drives; perhaps eating in S's case. Hammer (1980) also suggests that long necks may be drawn by those who have difficulty swallowing or psychogenic digestive disturbances. If this were present, this would only intensify her current digestive problems. The painting response is within Lowenfeld and Brittain's (1975) Schematic stage.

Clay Response

S then moved on to work with the clay. She began by verbally expressing ideas of great things to create, but had difficulty manipulating the stiff clay material. With assistance from the administrator, the client was able to roll the clay flat, which concluded in circular shape. S decided that she had made a pizza and began to add slices of pepperoni to the pizza. She cut herself a "slice," but remarked that it was gross because it was made from clay. Even

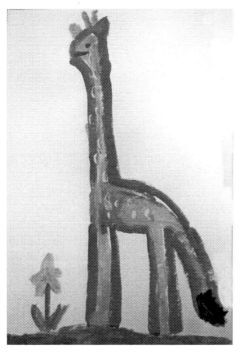

Figure 5.1. S's CATA Paint Response. (For color version, see Plate 4, p. 110.)

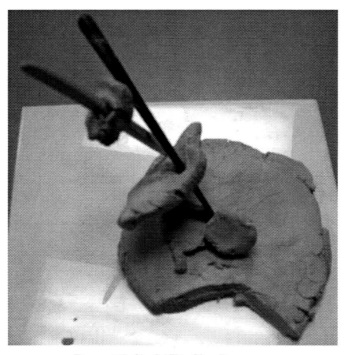

Figure 5.2. S's CATA Clay Response.

during play she is unable to escape her digestive reality. She then cut a second larger slice, which she drew a smiley face on; perhaps indicating the happiness that nonrestricted foods could bring. S regressed to stabbing the happy slice along with some of the pepperoni and the pizza itself, clearly displaying oral aggression. These actions are concurrent with her entering the session with wax Dracula teeth. S's clay response is within Lowenfeld and Brittain's (1975) Preschematic Stage. She quickly completed the clay portion and moved onto the pencil drawing, which she said "was best."

Draw Response

S began her pencil drawing by drawing a zebra. She had trouble deciding on the thickness of the zebra's neck but had no problem drawing the rest of the head and stripes. When she began the drawing S commented that she was only going to draw half of the zebra. S was also very confident about her ability to draw the zebra as she had "practiced a lot to become so good at drawing zebras." While doing her drawing, S told the administrator that she was "almost the smartest kid in her class" and that she "had been reading since she was four." Her desire to impress others may be an indication of a need for warmth and recognition. Once finished with the outline, S requested color pencils to fill in the zebra and its stripes; she even included the red hair that grows along the top of a zebra's mane. This may have been an attempt to display her knowledge, and again impress the administrator. Next she added the horse, which in comparison to the zebra, looks less practiced. Hammer (1980) suggests that a horse is often indicative of feeling as a helper or servant. Neither animal has a body, which could indicate a resort into fantasy, as well as, feelings of inferiority of body according to Hammer (1980); again S's body size is small for her age. S's drawing response was within Lowenfeld and Brittain's (1975) Schematic Stage.

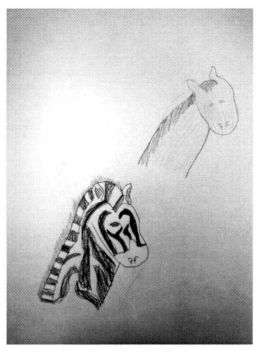

Figure 5.3. S's CATA Drawing Response. (For color version, see Plate 5, p. 111.)

Identified Patient: Lucy

DOB: August 25, 1978

CA: 28.2

Test Date: October 30, 2006

Administrant: Jordan M. Kroll

Assessment Administered: CATA

Refer to Appendix A for Genogram, Timeline, Behavioral Observations, and Psychosocial Indicators.

Draw Response

Sketching extremely lightly (image has been darkened for clarity) and tentatively, Lucy began to draw a building from a bird's-eye view, or, as she said, in an attempt to recall an "out of body" feeling. This perspective is quite unique, and quickly established her creative way of seeing everyday things. As she drew, Lucy's healthy perfectionism was hinted at as she asked, "Can you tell what it is yet?" Later, when she didn't know if she could accomplish an aspect of the drawing correctly, she asked for scrap paper to practice on. This tells of at least some investment in her creation and also of her desire to not ruin what she had already done. She was told that it was okay to erase, so she should go ahead and try her idea on the original drawing. She did so, was unsatisfied, and erased. Following this, Lucy began using the eraser end as much as the lead-end of the pencil, and also rotated the paper several different ways. Her difficulty seemed to be more a matter of depicting what she saw in her mind (mind/hand coordination) than of her hand and/or the pencil not being controlled properly (hand/eye coordination). After thirty-five minutes, Lucy had completed a semi-realistic drawing of a tall building on the corner of a city crossroads while being fairly successful in her admirable attempt at a difficult and fascinating perspective. The drawing, which covers the entire page, would probably be assessed at Lowenfeld & Brittain's (1975) Pseudo-Naturalistic Stage of development. Lucy showed great awareness of the environment, yet drew only the important elements (the building) in detail and was critical of her own shortcomings.

Clay Response

Lucy next put on a smock and grabbed a hunk of clay, which she played with somewhat aggressively for a few minutes, getting the feel for it. She first rolled it into a cone and from there formed a volcanic structure, which she readily smashed. Then she hollowed out a very rough bowl shape, using just her hands; but seeing that the bottom was too thin, she also destroyed this,

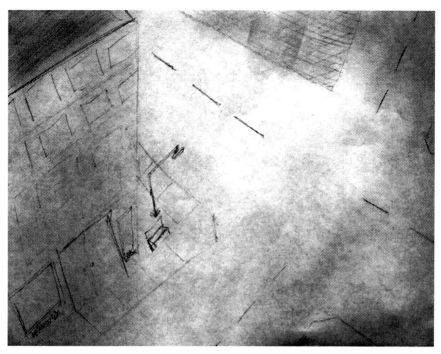

Figure 5.4. Lucy's CATA Drawing Response.

pounding the clay back into a solid mass. At this point, Lucy regressed to sensuously squishing the clay in both hands and giggling. Another attempt at a vessel, this time attaching the clay to the outside of a tin can, failed to produce desired results and Lucy stood up, laughing, perplexed, and stated, "I don't like this one." Yet her mind was still working through the dilemma, and it wasn't long before she began with renewed interest and energy. Another bowl was formed, mostly by hand until, learning from her previous efforts, she grabbed a yogurt container and pressed it into the bowl to give it a uniform shape and to make it "smooth and pretty." And thusly, she had transformed this ugly and frustrating lump of inanimate clay into something she found increasingly beautiful. She proceeded to cut the top flat with a metal tool and also to make a spoon accessory, stating that her creation was a Japanese bowl for miso soup. Lucy was now sitting back down and looking at her soup bowl proudly. She then said she was finished, only to decide a few seconds later that it needed decoration. Using a metal pick, she carved vine and leaf markings into it. Lucy's completed bowl and spoon represent creative problem solving and full reintegration after regression while working with the clay. This success seemed to pique Lucy's interest and excitement in art, and her demeanor for the remainder of the night reflected this newfound mastery.

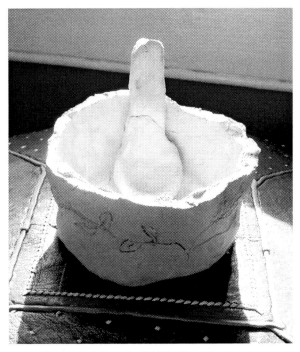

Figure 5.5. Lucy's CATA Clay Response.

Paint Response

It was evident as Lucy began to paint that she was more free and spontaneous in her approach, and the directive to "paint anything" was more easily accepted and not so overwhelming. She claimed to be familiar with the basics of mixing colors, but seemed new to it in practice. She chose two large brushes; with one added yellow to the turquoise, and with the other, brought red to that mix. "Aw, that's a cool color" was her response to the pale red-violet she had created. She then stood up and, choosing black, repetitiously painted long and curving strokes, covering a large portion of the vertically-oriented paper. Studies have shown that repetition in art can signify controlled, obsessive behavior or inhibition (Hammer, 1975), but could also mean healthy rhythm and fluidity. Perhaps, as in Lucy's case, both can exist simultaneously. The brushes she had used to mix were lying on the tray full of paint when she declared, "I need another fat brush." Here she remembered there was a cup of water in which to wash out her brushes, and utilized this. Still, she used four or five different brushes at once, balancing them on the tray between uses. Her addition of colors followed the pattern of the black as she layered them on top of each other. She didn't mix many colors in the tray; rather let them flow together and intermingle on the paper. The

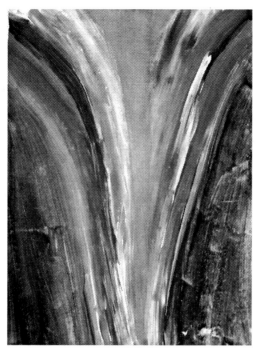

Figure 5.6. Lucy's CATA Paint Response. (For color version, see Plate 6, p. 111.)

many blues that dominate the colored area could represent energy according to Furth (Oster & Crone, 2004). White and the pale violet were added over the blues and greens, and eventually, most colors were included in the painting, as Lucy put on final touches of bold red and yellow highlights. Again, she stated that she was done, only to keep working and inquiring as to whether she could keep it. She titled it "Deep Calls unto Deep," which denotes the expression of a spiritual idea manifested in a new way. The colored section, resembling a waterfall that pours down the middle of the page, seems to dominate the black space or ground on either side of it. There is a balance of colors and an almost perfect vertical symmetry, which may allude to intrapersonal balance, yet may again reveal a controlling or perfecting personality (Hammer, 1975). The image is abstract and seems to pour off the page, possibly suggesting active imagination or fantasy life.

Conclusion

Lucy's CATA results present an ideal case to highlight personal learning and liberation through art. There was a definite turning point – an instant where suddenly, she was able to get in touch with and begin to express some of a wealth of long-dormant ideas by discovering new ways to utilize her inner resources and talents. Creative problem solving is surely one of these, and could be witnessed in action as she evolved from frustration and regression with the clay to completing a work of art that she was proud of and wanted to keep. In the other media, she experienced what it is to "lose oneself" in art as she progressed from a somewhat inhibited realism in drawing to a new realm of free and colorful abstraction while painting. Lucy has a unique vision of the world, and through this recent art experience, she has become inspired and excited at the new possibilities of self-expression.

Identified Patient: D

DOB: May 27, 1986

CA: 22

Testing Dates: September 28, 2007

Administrant: M. Trinidad Selman P.

Assessments Administered: CATA, KFD

See Chapter 8 for a further example regarding D.

Refer to Appendix A for Genogram, Timeline, Behavioral Observations, and Psychosocial Indicators.

Set-Up

The assessment was done in a quiet room at the library of Nazareth College, and it was illuminated only with artificial lights. Everything was thoroughly covered with newspapers in order not to interfere with the client's motivation to express freely with the different materials presented. All the materials were displayed on the table; recipient with different colors of acrylic painting, extra compartment for mixing colors, water, different kind of brushes, paper towel, white paper, clay, a piece of cardboard for the clay artwork, clay tools, a black pencil and an eraser.

Description and Behavioral Observations

D is a third-year undergraduate international student at Nazareth College of the International Studies program. She came to the U.S. on year 2005 from Nepal, where all her family lives. She visited her family on the summer of 2007 and it was supposed that she was not coming back because she had a problem with her U.S. Visa. Nonetheless, the problem was solved and she could come back. Yet in the confusion, she lost the living space she shared with some friends, (as she was not coming back) thus, she is staying temporarily at a professor's house until spring semester of 2007.

The whole assessment lasted 50 minutes. All the time, she was very cooperative; however, she seemed to be very anxious to the fact that she had to use art materials. Repeatedly she reported that she didn't know how to do it, and that the last time she picked up an art material was in elementary school.

Assessment Results

D was asked to choose one of the three possibilities of materials to work with: paints, clay or pencil. She immediately wanted to start with paints, in a manner to finish quickly. She stated "let's do this first, to finish with this as soon as possible." With this, the practitioner noted that she was very anxious. She was encouraged not to be afraid, and constantly the practitioner told her that nobody was going to grade her, that it was only an exercise and to try not to focus on the results.

Paint Response

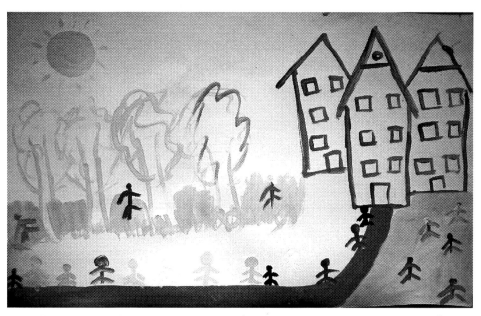

Figure 5.7. D's CATA Paint Response. (For color version, see Plate 7, p. 112.)

D started drawing the blue buildings saying that it was Nazareth College, specifically, Golisano Building, where she had almost all of her classes. She used turquoise to paint the environment, the grass, and trees. She commented that one of the things she liked most about Nazareth was the expansive green areas. She also stated that she liked turquoise. The people in the picture are students heading to class, and it was stated that it was a sunny and warm day. To paint the walkway to the building, she asked the practitioner to help her to make brown color. While painting, it seemed that her anxiety did not diminish, because she laughed about what she was doing. The quality of her artwork appeared to be very childish and stereotyped, with plain colors and line figures. She used the entire page and distributed the figures coherently. Form appeared to dominate color, representing a common scene of her life as a student. It seems that the artwork served as a defense over her anxiety; however, she brought part of her actual world, demonstrating with this that her studies and being without her family in another country, were important issues in her life. Her attitude in general was cooperative and anxious, as mentioned before, and with respect to her work, she manifested indifference. She exposed herself as uninterested in mixing colors, except for brown, and didn't put great effort on her work. The only occasion, in which she seemed to be enjoying work, was when she was using turquoise and painting the trees. The lines for them are the most free and loose of the entire picture. In regard to the developmental stage of painting, D used color and lines combined to represent a specific design. Green (turquoise) for trees and grass, brown for the walkway, yellow for the sun, blue for the buildings and all the same colors, including red, for all the people. Regarding to the facets of personality and the use of color, D had preference for cool colors, being the turquoise and blue predominant. She was very schematic and literal in representing a scene of her daily life. She didn't put emphasis in details and didn't use perspective. All these, indicate that she may be placed in a drawing stage level of a child, Schematic stage of development, age 7–9 years (Lowenfeld & Brittain, 1987).

Draw Response

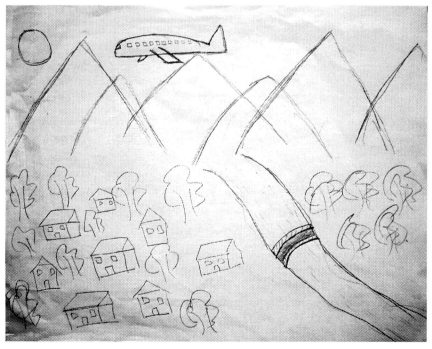

Figure 5.8. D's CATA Drawing Response.

For the second piece of work, D chose to draw. The picture is a landscape with an airplane, mountains, a river with a bridge and a kind of village. The drawing has an aerial perspective from above, as one would be situated at the same level of the plane. D described her drawing as her flying to Nepal to visit her home and family. This view between the mountains, just before landing, represents a little village near Katmandu, Nepal's capital city. She highlighted using pressure and lines in the airplane, mountains, river and bridge; however, she used very light and free lines in the village and trees. Hammer (1980) stated that variations in pressure correspond to individuals more flexible and adaptable, and that light and faint lines are seen in inadequate and depressed individuals. The same author (1980) indicated that a continuous line, frequently reinforced, is indicative of anxiety and insecurity. This supports what the practitioner perceived about D's attitude during the assessment. Hammer (1980) also describes meanings regarding the placement of the drawings. Although he explains different significances depending on the position of the whole drawing, the practitioner believes that the emphasis D gave in the different places of the drawing may also help to delineate her situation. If the drawing is placed above the mid-point of the page, it may reflect that the person is striving hard and that his goal is relatively unattainable and that the subject tends to seek satisfaction in fantasy rather than in reality (Hammer, 1980). If the drawing is placed below the mid-point of the page, this may indicate that the "subject feels insecure and inadequate, and that this feeling is producing a depression of mood" (Hammer, 1980, p. 70). Looking at D's drawing, one can relate the emphasis given in the upper side of the page, in the mountains and airplane, as something unattainable. D's desire to go to Nepal and visit her family is not an option for now. The light lines and the placement of houses and trees in the lower part of the page, are both signs that may indicate that she is developing depression symptoms. At this moment of the assessment, on one hand D seemed to be more relaxed; but on the other hand, she still repeated "This is very childish," and asked "Who is going to see this?", indicating that she was guarded. The practitioner had to reassure D that her identity would not be revealed. Regarding the developmental stage of the artwork, D made a spatial representation of the landscape using visual perspective. This was different from her first artwork, in which she did not use perspective as a visual resource. In regard to signs of constitutional problems, D presented as having no problem with form, perception, fine motor control, or coordination. Finally, on the subject of facets of personality, she used the entire page, and the size of the mountains in relation to the airplane; houses and trees appear out of proportion. The airplane should appear smaller, the same as the houses and trees. In spite of this, the whole drawing is very coherent and reaches the objective of showing an aerial view, as D was above the airplane about to land. The theme was personal; but the way in which she drew the village (houses and trees) was banal. For a second time, the practitioner perceived D's concern of being far away from home.

Clay Response

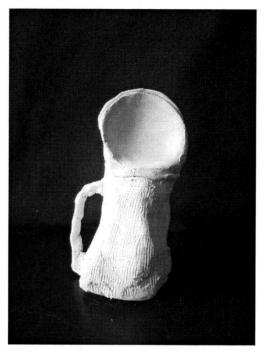

Figure 5.9. D's CATA Clay Response. (20 cm. [height] x 5 cm. [diameter] aprox.)

When D finally realized that clay was the last material to work with, she again displayed anxiety, saying "I don't know what to do. I haven't used clay since my elementary school days!" The practitioner encouraged her to let the clay show her a form. Again, I suggested that she not be concerned about the results. She started by squeezing the piece of clay, and while she repeated "What can I do?" she stroked it, and started giving it a rather phallic form. Finally, she stated "This is only an object for decoration." The practitioner asked her if there was a place for it somewhere. D suggested that the garden would be a good place for it. She would put a mirror in the round space to reflect the sun and situate it in some place to maintain it, always illuminated. Finally, she expressed that it would be an object to put in her mother's garden; thus, she would keep it until she goes back to Nepal, because here there is no place that really belongs to her. Once more, D expressed her desire to be with her family in her home country, and the feeling of "not belonging."

In regard to the developmental stage of clay modeling, D was able to construct an abstract object from a whole piece of clay and to stick together two pieces. She used both hands to work and did not have a problem with her hands becoming dirty. In general, she enjoyed working with clay although she did not know what to do.

Discussion

Oster and Crone (2004) describe developmental progressions mentioning different authors to complement the information, such as Gardner, Lowenfeld and Brittain, and Kellogg among others. Furthermore, Horovitz (2007) states that an adult can be placed in one of the different stages of drawings described for children between one and 17 years old. According to this, D could be placed between the Schematic stage (7–9 years old) and the Gang stage (10–12 years old; Lowenfeld & Brittain, 1987). The reason for this can be seen in both 2D artworks, in which are very schematic representations. One can see enough details to recognize what she wanted to represent; but at the same time, she is not interested in details. D was able to depict her environment in a literal way (Oster & Crone, 2004).

Comparing all three artworks, there were no similarities besides the schematic and literality of the way of drawing. However, the practitioner may state that the similarities were more in the way that D worked, her attitude in front of the art materials, and her verbalizations while working. The themes that appear were in some kind of order. In the first artwork, D got connected with the actual moment of her life as a student. In the second artwork, she thought about where she would like to be (Nepal and with her family). Finally, she made an object to keep until she returns to Nepal, suggesting a desire for belonging. This object could represent her feeling of expectation to achieve that goal. The lack of details in D's artworks may also indicate that D is having feelings of emptiness and reduced energy, suggesting depressive symptoms (Hammer, 1980). This issue, in addition to the light lines of the second artwork, might indicate depression of mood, and might suggest her desire for support and assistance. This was also concertized by D's verbalizations, making references to the difficulty of being far from home, her friends (loss of her space in the department), and to the fact that she is living with a woman in a place where she doesn't feel comfortable.

Identified Patient: Sandy

DOB: May 23, 1972

CA: 33

Testing Date: April 9, 2006

Administrant: Rachel N. Sikorski

Assessments Administered: CATA, FSA, PPAT

See Chapters 6 and 9 for further examples regarding Sandy.

Refer to Appendix A for Genogram, Timeline, Behavioral Observations, and Psychosocial Indicators.

Clay Response

For the CATA assessment, Sandy was given the choice to draw, paint or sculpt something out of clay. Although Sandy stated that she had little experience with clay, this medium was her enthusiastic first choice. Sandy worked quickly and quietly, and appeared to be deeply engaged while completing this response. The clay was squeezed and pulled into differentiated shapes, which were then stuck together to form a two-dimensional flower. With this, Sandy was able to make a successful attempt at formed expression (Horovitz-Darby, 1988). Sandy appeared highly invested in her work, but as demonstrated in previous assessments (see Chapter 6 and Chapter 9), her attitude toward her artwork remained the same as she commented on its low quality. Sandy's ability to work additively with the clay and add superficial details to her creation places her at the Gang Age Stage of development (9–12 years), according to Lowenfeld and Brittain (1985).

Paint Response

During the CATA paint response, Sandy told the writer how uncomfortable she was with the lack of structure for the art tasks. Despite this lack of structure, the writer observed Sandy express herself most freely during this response. Unlike her responses to the other art assessments (see Chapter 6 and Chapter 9), Sandy appeared to work slower, more thoughtfully, and expressed herself with more color while painting. The writer observed Sandy's experimental play with the paint result in a successful attempt at formed expression (Horovitz-Darby, 1988). Sandy created a bright, flower-like pattern that appeared similar in theme to the clay response. After the painting was complete, Sandy expressed that she would have liked to use purple in her response. When the writer inquired as to why Sandy chose not

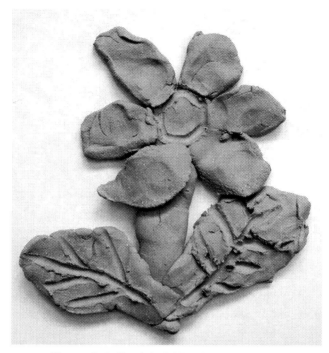

Figure 5.10. Sandy's CATA Clay Response.

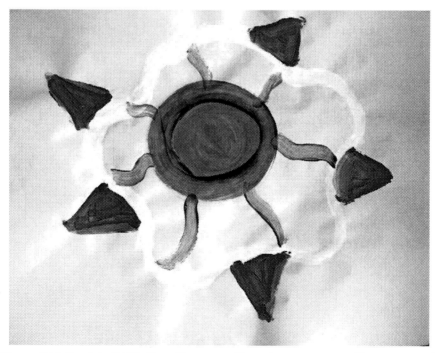

Figure 5.11. Sandy's CATA Paint Response. (For color version, see Plate 8, p. 112.)

to mix the desired color, she explained that she never thought of it. This oversight may be a reflection of Sandy's lack of confidence or inexperience with the materials. Sandy's CATA paint response puts her at the Schematic Stage (7–9 years) of development, according to Lowenfeld and Brittain (1985).

Draw Response

The final response of the session was the CATA drawing. Sandy's picture was done very quickly, with light pressure and a scribble-like line quality. This may indicate anxiety, a minimal effort to comply with the task, or lack of confidence in regard to the medium (Hammer, 1980). There is a large sun shining in the upper right-hand corner of the page, which may reflect the potential need for warmth and support (Burns & Kaufman, 1972). The flowers and tree in Sandy's picture are lined up on a baseline. This spatial representation, as well as the line quality and use of representational objects or symbols in her drawing place Sandy between the Preschematic (4–7 years) and Schematic (7–9 years) stages of development (Lowenfeld & Brittain, 1985).

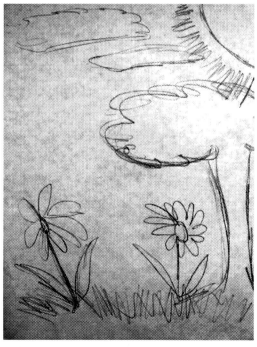

Figure 5.12. Sandy's CATA Drawing Response.

Conclusion

Sandy was invested in her work on the three CATA responses; however, she spent little time working and depicted only minimal details. Sandy's attitude toward her artwork seemed to remain constant during the session, as she often used sarcasm when commenting on the quality of her responses. She expressed enjoyment and a preference for working with clay and paint after completing the CATA assessment; mediums with which Sandy would produce her most creative expressions of the session. Overall, Sandy's responses to the CATA assessments place her at the Schematic (7–9 years) stage of development, according to Lowenfeld and Brittain (1985).

Recommendations and Conclusion

Sandy's responses to the FSA (see Chapter 6), PPAT (see Chapter 9) and CATA assessments may reflect anxiety, a lack of confidence and a distorted self-perception. Her family history and experience as the middle child of her family may have had an impact on her self-concept and confidence.

Sandy's expressions are simple, reserved, and quickly executed. Her role as middle child in the family, as well as her experiences of receiving less attention than her siblings, may have influenced her self-perception. The building of creativity and the promotion of self-expression that art therapy offers may be beneficial for Sandy in developing increased self-knowledge and more confidence in her abilities.

The writer recommends that Sandy consider engaging in art therapy on a regular basis, so that she may find a constructive outlet for emotional expression and develop increased self-confidence and a stronger self-concept.

Chapter 6

FACE STIMULUS ASSESSMENT (FSA)

INTRODUCTION

Donna Betts

The Face Stimulus Assessment (FSA; Betts, 2003) is a standardized projective drawing assessment designed for use with individuals from multicultural backgrounds with multiple disabilities, communication disorders, and autism. The FSA has been used with other client populations, for example Russian orphans (Robb, 2001) and a normative college population (Hamilton & Betts, 2008).

The FSA is comprised of a series of three pieces of white 8.5" x 11" paper: Picture 1 consists of a standardized image of a human face; Picture 2 contains an outline of the face only, and Picture 3 is a blank page. Additional materials include a standard packet of eight Crayola© markers, and a packet of eight Crayola© Multicultural markers. The markers are mixed randomly and placed on a table where the test is administered. The FSA can be conducted individually or in a group setting. The assessment directive is simple: "Use the markers and this piece of paper." After the client completes Picture 1, it is removed completely from his or her view, and replaced with Picture 2. Following completion of Picture 2, it is removed from the client's view and replaced with Picture 3, the blank piece of paper, in vertical format. The administrator is encouraged to review the assessment with the client as follow-up.

Until recently, the rating method for the FSA consisted of informal guidelines (Betts, 2008). However, Michelle Hamilton, who at the time of this writing is a master's candidate in art therapy at Avila University, conducted her thesis on the establishment of a standardized rating system for the FSA. Hamilton and Betts (2008) adapted nine of the 14 scales from the Formal

Elements Art Therapy Scale (FEATS; Gantt & Tabone, 1998) to rate the second picture in the FSA series. Thirty drawings from a normative sample of college students were used in this study. Nine of the 14 FEATS scales were adapted to rate the FSA drawing: #1, Prominence of Color; #2, Color Fit; #3, Implied Energy; #6, Logic; #7, Realism; #9, Developmental Level; #10, Details of Objects and Environment; #11, Line Quality; #14, Perseveration. This was possible because the FEATS is adaptable for rating other types of artwork (Anschela, Dolceb, Schwartzmanc, & Fishera, 2005; Gantt, 2001; Swan-Foster, N., Foster, S., & Dorsey, A., 2003). Further validity and reliability studies are needed in order to establish the FSA as a sound instrument, but the Hamilton and Betts research is a step in the right direction. This study can be built upon to further justify use of the nine adapted FEATS scales for rating drawing number 2 of the FSA.

The present chapter presents two case studies using the FSA. The first depicts the FSA of "Pam," a 54-year-old woman with traumatic brain injury. The second case study illustrates the FSA pictures of "Sandy." For both of these cases, the informal rating procedure from the FSA Guidelines (Betts, 2008) was used to formulate possible interpretations of the drawings.

More information about the FSA is available on Donna Betts' website, http://www.art-therapy.us/FSA.htm.

Identified Patient: Pam

DOB: August, 1954

CA: 52

Testing Dates: September 27, 2006; March 21, 2007; March 28, 2007

Administrant: Julie Riley

Assessments Administered: BATA, FSA, SDT

See Chapters 3 and 10 for further examples regarding Pam.

Refer to Appendix A for Genogram, Timeline, Behavioral Observations, and Psychosocial Indicators.

Despite Pam's impairment due to the TBI (see Appendix A), she made serious attempts to stay inside the lines. She asked if she could "erase" or "wipe off" the marker, which implies she cognitively understood the line's purpose despite her inaccurate manual dexterity. Before the TBI, Pam was left-handed but now uses her right hand due to left hemiparesis, (which is still a point of struggle for her). Pam took approximately half an hour for the first face assessment template before prompted to move on to the second tem-

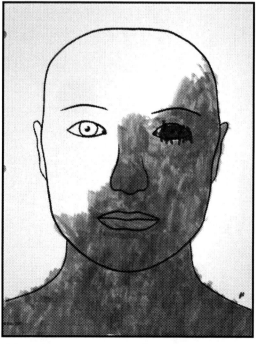

Figure 6.1. Pam's SDT Picture 1 Response. (For color version, see Plate 9, p. 113.)

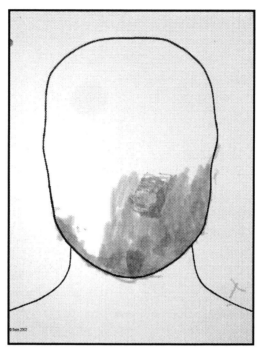

Figure 6.2. Pam's SDT Picture 2 Response. (For color version, see Plate 10, p. 113.)

plate, which she worked on for 15 minutes. Due to the lack of boundaries available for the third phase, she struggled to begin for seven minutes and questioned this writer regarding what she should draw. According to Pam she decided to draw "a person's head because I was really good at those before my accident." All she could complete before the session ended was the beginnings of a "hair flip." Throughout the stimulus drawings, she used appropriate colors: dark tan or beige for skin (see Plate 9 and Plate 10), red for lips (see Plate 9), brown for the eye (see Plate 9), brown for the hair (see Plate 11). Product completion focused on the right side of the paper is consistent with perceptual difficulties as a result of brain injury. "Visual Inattention, commonly associated with injuries to the right hemisphere, usually involves lack of awareness of visual stimuli in the left visual field" (Cheyne-King, 1990, p. 69). This might also reflect emotional instability as Hammer suggests, "drawings which display an obvious lack of symmetry have been found to indicate equivalent inadequate feelings of security in the subject's emotional life" (Hammer, 1980, p. 68).

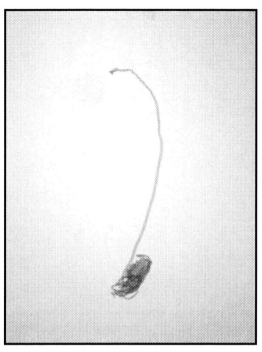

Figure 6.3. Pam's SDT Picture 3 Response. (For color version, see Plate 11, p. 114.)

Identified Patient: Sandy

DOB: May 23, 1972

CA: 33

Testing Date: April 9, 2006

Administrant: Rachel N. Sikorski

Assessments Administered: CATA, FSA, PPAT

See Chapters 5 and 9 for further examples regarding Sandy.

Refer to Appendix A for Genogram, Timeline, Behavioral Observations, and Psychosocial Indicators.

Sandy responded to the first directive, "Use these markers and this piece of paper" by asking, "I can do what I want? Okay!" She seemed enthusiastic about working on the first picture and began to work by using a brown marker to enlarge the eyebrows of the face. Sandy made it a point to state this and many subsequent actions to the writer as she worked. Sandy chose a red-orange marker to draw hair next, and as she colored it in, she stated aloud that this picture would be a self-portrait. With that, Sandy set down the marker she was using and touched her hand to her face. She seemed to be searching for the pockmark on her left cheek; and as it was discovered, Sandy proceeded to depict it in her picture using a black marker. Sandy's decision to indicate a flaw on the face of her "self-portrait" may point to the possibility of poor self-esteem or a distorted self-perception (Betts, 2004). Sandy continued to work on the picture by coloring in the lips with peach, the eyes with light brown, and some eyelashes with black. She looked through the markers to find a color for the skin, but could not decide on one. The writer made an attempt to assist Sandy, but she decided that the face did not need to be colored.

The second drawing was administered with the same directive as the first, to which Sandy responded by laughing and stating, "I don't know what I'm doing!" It seemed to this writer that Sandy was anxious and may have wanted to have more structure or direction about what to draw. Sandy delayed for a few seconds before using black to quickly depict eyes, a nose, a mouth, and two ears. The eyes appear to be slightly crossed, which could be an indicator of Sandy's potential inability to focus on her environment. Lastly, Sandy used red to draw and color in a tongue-like shape above the mouth. She laughed as she added this final detail, and finished by stating: "This is a masterpiece – the Louvre!" The addition of a tongue sticking out may suggest rebellion or obstinacy, even though Sandy complied with the drawing task.

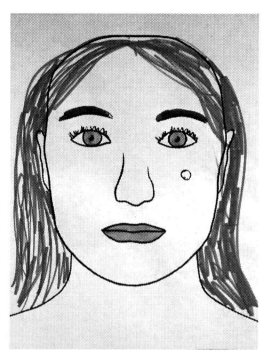

Figure 6.4. Sandy's SDT Picture 1 Response. (For color version, see Plate 12, p. 114.)

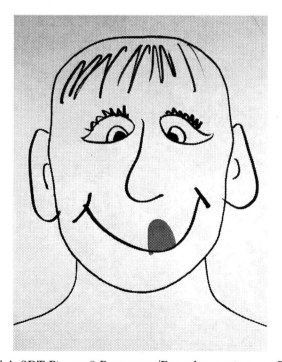

Figure 6.5. Sandy's SDT Picture 2 Response. (For color version, see Plate 13, p. 115.)

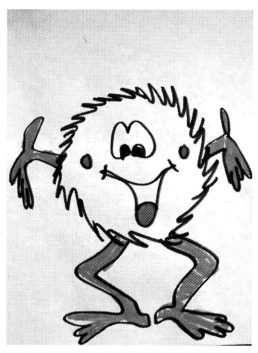

Figure 6.6. Sandy's SDT Picture 3 Response. (For color version, see Plate 14, p. 115.)

It can be seen in this second drawing that Sandy left the face and background white, and limited her color choices to black and red only. This limited use of color could be an indicator of anxiety and may reflect some concern in reference to performing the drawing task "correctly," or in a way that would please the administrator. Moreover, the second picture does not appear to be similar to Sandy's first, which was more naturalistic and labeled a "self-portrait." Instead, the second picture seems most likely to be a representation of Sandy's attitude, rather than an actual person. The attitude is one of denigrating humor and the product in the service of defense, as indicated by the red, stuck-out tongue, slight cross-eyes and Sandy's sarcastic comment about the picture's quality (The Louvre).

Sandy completed the final FSA drawing by depicting a large, jagged-edged circle with facial features. The face of the character created was given rosy-red cheeks and a red tongue; its arms and legs were colored in quickly with orange. She described this character as a "doodle," and told the writer that doodling is something that she enjoys doing whenever she is bored. Sandy's decision to draw something other than a face seemed to be a creative, rather than rebellious, artistic choice (Betts, 2004). When looking at the final picture, one can see that the line quality of the central, circular form and the color within the character's arms and legs appears to be sketchy. This, in conjunction with Sandy's quick response and safe color choices – as seen in pictures one and two – could be another indicator of anxiety or a lack of confidence.

Recommendations and Conclusion

Sandy's responses to the FSA, PPAT (see Chapter 9) and CATA (see Chapter 5) assessments may reflect anxiety, a lack of confidence and a distorted self-perception. Her family history and experience as the middle child of her family may have had an impact on her self-concept and confidence.

Sandy's expressions are simple, reserved, and quickly executed. Her role as middle child in the family, as well as her experiences of receiving less attention than her siblings, may have influenced her self-perception. The building of creativity and the promotion of self-expression that art therapy offers may be beneficial for Sandy in developing increased self-knowledge and more confidence in her abilities.

The writer recommends that Sandy consider engaging in art therapy on a regular basis, so that she may find a constructive outlet for emotional expression and develop increased self-confidence and a stronger self-concept.

Chapter 7

HOUSE-TREE-PERSON ASSESSMENT (HTP)

According to Buck (1966) and Hammer (1980), when a person draws the House, Tree and Person (in the HTP [House-Tree-Person] test), it is a reflection of the subject's inner view of his or her environment, the things that he or she considers of importance, as well as the self. The subtests of the HTP are saturated with symbolic, emotional and ideational experiences linked to personality development; therefore, the drawings of these images drive projection of the drawer. Developmentally, the favorite drawing object of young children has been touted as the human figure, followed by the house, and then the tree (Griffiths, 1935). Moreover, according to Rivière (1950), when children built with blocks, he discovered that construction was capable of symbolizing the child's body, a womb, and the parental home. (However, it is important to note that "empirical data of the HTP drawings supported the first and third of these symbolic meanings more frequently than the second" [Hammer, 1980, p. 167].) Rivière (1950) established that anomalies in the construction of the house building were synonymous with the alterations in the body image, which was later confirmed by Buck (1966). Indeed, the perception of the human being has been correlated to the saturated, emotive experiences associated with an individual's growth (Machover, 1949; Buck, 1966; Levy, 1950). Hammer (1980) reported the following: the house (as a dwelling place) arouses associations of home life and intra-familial relationships and both the tree and the person tap into the core personality of both body image and self-concept. (Specifically, the tree seems to reveal the more unconscious aspects of the subject, including the environmental life force. The person conveys the closer to conscious view of the subject and the relationship with the environment.) Hammer (1980) went one step further. He suggested: (1) the roof of the house to be equivalent to the blossom of the tree and the head of the person; (2) the body of the house to be correspondent to the body of the tree and person; and finally (3) the base of the house to be equivalent to the root of the tree and feet of the person. When viewed from this positioning, interesting parallels from the dissimilar subtests indeed strengthen the core premise underlying this projective tool.

While the authors will not cover all of the specific interpretations of the HTP, the editors redirect the reader to the Hammer (1980) text for an indepth review of these variables. Administration of the subtests will be reviewed before the presentation of the case samples that follow.

Although the subject is asked to draw a House, a Tree, and a Person, he or she is *not* told what kind of house, tree, or person to draw. Since clues do not generate from the examiner, the subject's response: size, type, placement, age, sex, facial expression, race, clothing, presentation (side, three-quarter, rear, or full view) are some examples of variations that can occur within the subtests. The subject is given a number two pencil with eraser and is employed to draw first achromatically a House, a Tree, and a Person. While the original test employs a four-form sheet of white paper (7.5 x 8 inches), in past years, clinicians have used a traditional 8.5" x 11" white paper. It is important to place the sheet horizontally when requesting the subject's rendition of the House and presented the paper vertically when requiring the Tree and Person. If the subject alters the direction of the paper, this can be duly noted by the administrant. The subject is then informed to draw any kind of House, Tree, or Person and to take as much time as he or she needs to complete the assessment. Drawings should be done freehand and without the use of a ruler or similar drawing tool. The order of presentation of the stimuli always remains consistent: House, then Tree, and then Person (Hammer, 1980, p. 166). When employing the chromatic version of the HTP, the assessment tool incorporates the same administration (as above) but eliminating the pencil and using Crayola© crayons with only eight colors: red, green, yellow, blue, brown, black, purple, and orange (Hammer, 1980, p. 209). Hammer (1980) contends that the chromatic HTP "cuts through the defenses to bare a deeper level of personality than does the achromatic set of drawings" (p. 208). The subject is allowed to use any or all of the eight crayons and can employ corrective measures as best able with the rudimentary aspects of the crayon. Post-drawing interrogation (of achromatic and chromatic subtests) by the clinician can further illuminate the emotive concerns of the subject. It is recommended that the drawings be developmentally categorized for cognitive levels of function, utilizing scales by Horovitz (2002) and/or Lowenfeld (1985).

Identified Patient: Holly

DOB: 1978

CA: 27

Testing Dates: April 2, 2006

Administrant: Jane C. Adams

Assessments Administered: ATDA, HTP, PPAT

See Chapters 2 and 9 for further examples regarding Holly.

Refer to Appendix A for Genogram, Timeline, Behavioral Observations, and Psychosocial Indicators.

The information in Holly's timeline may indicate that she struggles with intimacy and that she possibly has privacy issues (see Appendix A). Holly described experiences and behavior that seem to indicate the presence of anxiety as a constant in her life. She wrote of a new elementary school experience resulting in vomiting daily. Holly's unmet need for attention at home was noted as she commented on her sisters' psychological problems. Holly's drawings for the House-Tree-Person (HTP) assessment may validate her intimacy and privacy issues. She appears to be conflicted between her desire to open up to contact or intimacy with others and her fear that she may not receive the attention or approval that she craves. Her documented family experiences may show that she has repeatedly had to compete for attention in an unstable environment. The outcomes of these may have taught her that she cannot trust. According to Oster and Crone (2004), details such as shrubs "indicate a need to ground or structure her environment more completely and may be associated with a need to exercise control in interpersonal contact." Every window and shutter in Holly's house subtest appears wide-open. Hammer (1980) and Oster and Crone (2004) interpret open windows as a desire for outside contact. Open shutters may be indicators of a desire to control interaction with the environment including interpersonal relationships. Hammer (1980) further suggests that this results in anxiety and exhibits as nonconfrontational interaction.

House

Holly has drawn her house from a "worm's-eye view," looking up the front steps toward an apparently imposing entry. This perspective may express feelings of an unattainable, yet desirable home life. These feelings may be based on low self-esteem or a perception of unworthiness, even rejection or inferiority (Hammer, 1980, p. 178). In her chromatic HTP house sub-

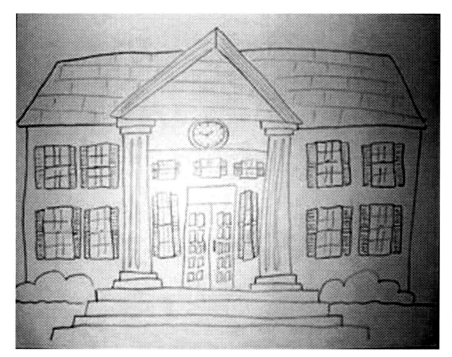

Figure 7.1. Holly's HTP Achromatic House.

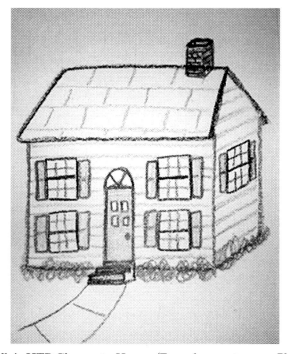

Figure 7.2. Holly's HTP Chromatic House. (For color version, see Plate 15, p. 116.)

test, Holly drew the house from an elevated perspective. This view has been interpreted as a rejection of the familial situation (Hammer, 1980). The difference between her house subtests appears to be primarily in the presentation of Holly's own rejection of the family situation in the chromatic version versus her apparent assumption of being rejected in the achromatic. Additional support for this view of rejection in the achromatic house drawing is denoted by the absence of the chimney, which was present in Holly's chromatic version. Oster and Crone (2004) suggest that a chimney may be representational of warmth. The missing chimney may further substantiate Holly's assumption of familial rejection.

Tree

Achromatic drawing tends to represent what the artist wants to be (Brooke, 2004). In Holly's tree subtest, she continues to illustrate her possible desire for outside contact that was noticed with the open windows in the house subtest. The tree branches grow out to the side of the page possibly reaching out to others and showing her desired interaction with her environment. But the tree also grows off the top of the page possibly indicating a retreat into fantasy (Hammer, 1980). Holly's chromatic tree branches are more vertical and reach more directly toward a mental life.

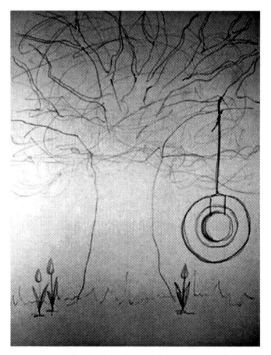

Figure 7.3. Holly's HTP Achromatic Tree.

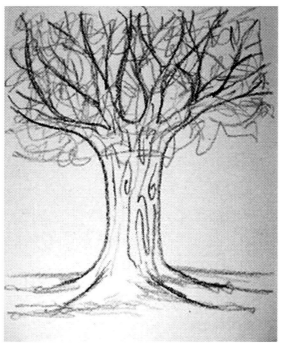

Figure 7.4. Holly's HTP Chromatic Tree. (For color version, see Plate 16, p. 116.)

A possibly significant difference between Holly's two drawings is the presence of roots in the chromatic drawing and their absence in the achromatic drawing. According to Oster and Crone (2004), a ground line present with no visible roots may indicate repressed emotions. Holly continues to present her apparent conflict between intimacy and a desire for connection with others in her tree subtests.

Person

In both of Holly's person subtests, she places emphasis on the head and face. The head is quite large in proportion to the body. Oster and Crone (2004) interpret this as a preoccupation with fantasy or mental life. They also note that the person drawing indicates conscious awareness of body image and self-concept both physically and psychologically (Oster & Crone, 2004). Both drawings bear a strong resemblance to Holly. In the chromatic drawing, the person is seated in a chair but in the achromatic version, the figure seems to be floating, not grounded on the page. Both figures show Holly's further preoccupation with fantasy in that the proportions allow the feet to disappear off the bottom of the page due to the sizing of the head. Both fig-

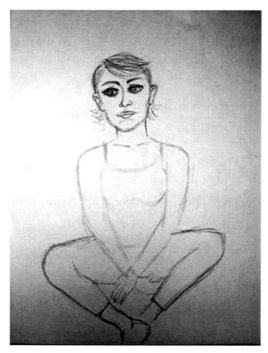

Figure 7.5. Holly's HTP Achromatic Person.

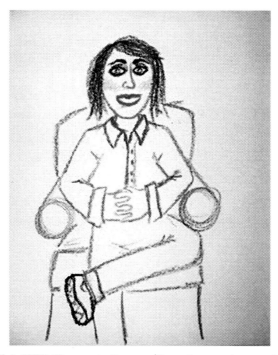

Figure 7.6. Holly's HTP Chromatic Person. (For color version, see Plate 17, p. 117.)

ures' arms are held close to their bodies possibly reinforcing the repressed emotions noted by the lack of roots in the tree subtest (Hammer, 1980; Oster & Crone, 2004).

Conclusion

It seems to this writer that Holly struggles with conflict and anxiety. She appears to be conflicted between her desire to reach out to others and to her environment versus her preoccupation with her own fantasy or mental life and an associated need for privacy. Holly may suffer from fear of intimacy as indicated by her HTP results. Her apparent need to repress her emotions and utilize tact in interacting with others rather than expressing her internal feelings, may be adding to Holly's anxiety. Her timeline shows an unstable home-life existed for a prolonged period. Holly felt she did not receive the attention she needed from her family. This is also reflected in her house sub-tests and would seem to contribute to her long-standing anxieties. Her House-Tree-Person (HTP) drawings show that Holly is in Horovitz's (2002) Artistic Developmental Stage.

Identified Patient: Diane

DOB: June 5, 1962

CA: 44

Testing Date: October 14, 2006; October 18, 2006

Administrant: Day Butcher

Assessments Administered: HTP

Refer to Appendix A for Genogram, Timeline, Behavioral Observations, and Psychosocial Indicators.

Diane's chromatic and achromatic series of drawings look very similar with only slight difference such as placement, summer/fall theme, or clothing of the person. Each drawing was made in a hurried fashion; she didn't put much time or thought into any of the six drawings, with the exception of the person drawings. As seen in each of the six drawings there is a key element of the bottom of the paper being the foundation and having to eliminate the girl's feet for lack of room. The relationship of the drawn subject such as the house with regard to the ground level indicates the person's relationship with reality. For example, a schizophrenic person may draw a house floating over the ground line and would not have a firm footing on reality (Hammer, 1980). In Diane's case not drawing a ground line may not indicate that she doesn't have a firm hold on reality, as she displays no signs of this diagnosis, but that she displays vulnerability to stressors (Oster & Crone, 2004). The trees having been drawn with the ground as the bottom edge of the paper is also representational that she may not have adequate feelings and by "clinging" to the bottom of the page indicated her need for security (Hammer, 1980). This feeling of inadequacy may also be revealed in her need to place accessories around the house in the form of a tree, sun, and grass (Hammer, 1980).

House

Looking further into the details of the house, Diane may display her willingness to receive people through the double doors of her drawn house. Diane also conveys this desire for outside contact and openness by filling the house with windows (Oster & Crone, 2004). On the other hand, by drawing the windows bare with no curtains, shutters, or cross lines her "interact[ion] with those in the environment [is] in an overly blunt and direct fashion" (Hammer, 1980, p. 177; Oster & Crone, 2004). Another aspect of the house that should be taken into consideration is that Diane included a chimney

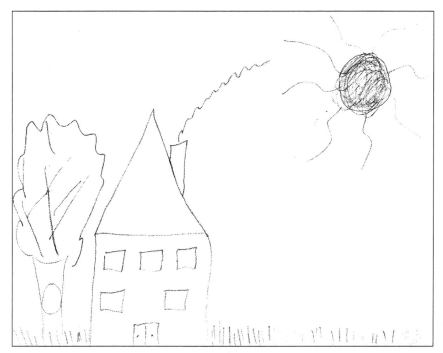

Figure 7.7. Diane's HTP Achromatic House.

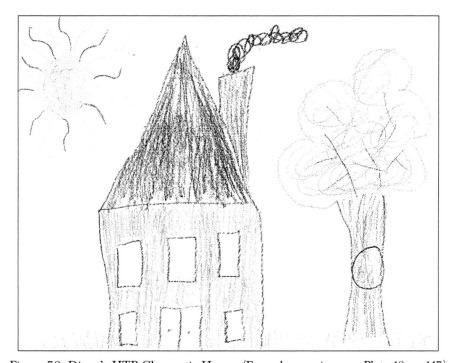

Figure 7.8. Diane's HTP Chromatic House. (For color version, see Plate 18, p. 117.)

with smoke coming out of it, which conveys warmth and affection (Oster & Crone, 2004). The smoke dramatically blowing in one direction, as seen in the chromatic house, may be indicative of the environmental pressures Diane feels, for example expressing the need to become employed or her sobriety from alcohol (Hammer, 1980).

Tree

In looking into the drawings of the tree, each represents different seasons, the achromatic being spring or summer and the chromatic of the current season fall. Each of the trees she drew both in the tree portion and those included with the house include a knothole. The knothole can signify some type of trauma in her life (Hammer, 1980; Oster & Crone, 2004). The knothole in each tree is placed in the center of the trunk, which may indicate that the trauma happened in middle adulthood. This trauma may signify her alcoholism and need to begin attendance at Alcohol Anonymous.

Person

Diane took a little bit more time and care in drawing the two girls one in which she identifies as her daughter, achromatic, and the other, chromatic, although very similar in looks was not. The achromatic girl was drawn with dimples and without her two top front teeth and long hair portraying the looks of her 8-year-old daughter. Therefore, the bearing of teeth, which usually symbolized aggression, should be disregarded in Diane's case. However, by drawing the girls with large broad shoulders, Diane displays her preoccupation with the need for strength (Oster & Crone, 2004).

Conclusion

Diane's chromatic and achromatic series of drawings look very similar with only slight difference such as placement, summer/fall theme, and clothing of the person. Diane's inability to move in or control her environment, insecurity, and vulnerability may be represented in the series of drawings, indicative of the paper edge as the baseline being the foundation for the trees and houses and having eliminated the girl's feet. These environmental pressures may include her expression of the need to find a part-time job and sobriety difficulties. Although, Diane was initially insecure about drawing the images of the house, tree, and person, art therapy may be an appropriate means to explore these insecurities and exploration of gaining control.

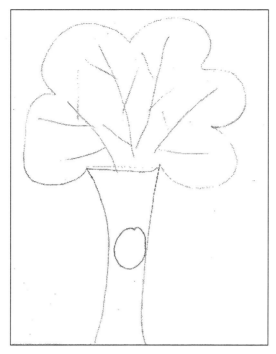

Figure 7.9. Diane's HTP Achromatic Tree.

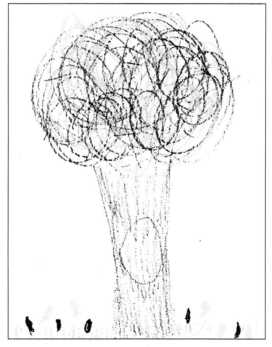

Figure 7.10. Diane's HTP Chromatic Tree. (For color version, see Plate 19, p. 118.)

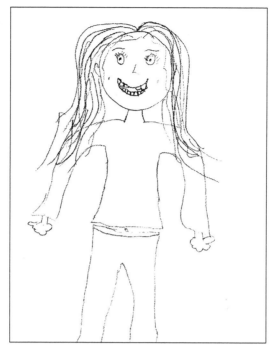

Figure 7.11. Diane's HTP Achromatic Person.

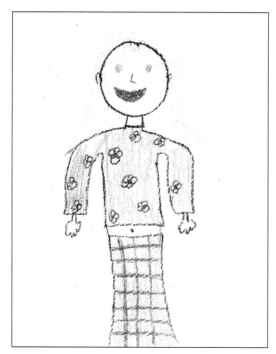

Figure 7.12. Diane's HTP Chromatic Person. (For color version, see Plate 20, p. 118.)

Identified Patient: Karen

DOB: December 17, 1982

CA: 22

Testing Date: October 6, 2005

Administrant: Rachel N. Sikorski

Assessments Administered: HTP

Refer to Appendix A for Genogram, Timeline, Behavioral Observations, and Psychosocial Indicators.

Achromatic House

Karen responded to the house directive by drawing a very large rectangle, topped by a wide triangle. She added three horizontal lines that extend from the top, middle, and base of the house to the left edge of the page. Because she drew such large shapes on a piece of paper that was vertically oriented, the house seems to extend beyond the border of the drawing page. This suggests poor planning, and is likely a sign of Karen's lack of artistic confidence. The house seems to cling to the edge of the paper, which might reflect a need for support, fear of independent action, and/or a lack of self-assurance (Hammer, 1980).

Karen continued by adding a number of details to the house: four small windows, one large window, a front door, and a garage door. The presence of several windows might express Karen's desire for outside contact. Nevertheless, clear crosses or bars through the windows could signify a need for controlled interaction with the environment (Hammer, 1980). The front door was placed on the baseline of the house, yet Karen did not create a path leading up to the house. Along with the small size of the door, this omission once again underscores a need for security by limiting or controlling access (Hammer, 1980). Karen did not depict a ground line for the house, and therefore may have been communicating feelings of instability in reference to her family situation. The absence of a chimney might indicate a lack of psychological warmth in the household and may possibly represent Karen's desire for understanding and acceptance from her mother (Oster & Crone, 2004). This is something Karen may have felt she did not receive after younger sister, Kelly, was born.

Despite lacking confidence in her drawing skills, Karen's depiction constituted an attempt to create a three-dimensional representation of a house that she later identified as her first home. Since most subjects tend to choose the house (or tree or person) that harbors affinity or identification, it seems like-

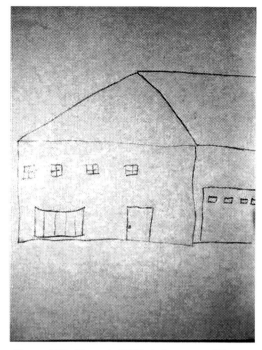

Figure 7.13. Karen's HTP Achromatic House.

ly that Karen's depiction illustrates her perception of, or unconscious feelings about, the instability within her home environment (Hammer, 1980).

Achromatic Tree

The next task completed by Karen was the drawing of a tree. This drawing took Karen less than one minute to execute, and when finished, she looked at the writer and giggled. She communicated a lack of confidence in her artistic ability and disappointment in her drawing by stating, "It's a sad-looking tree." Karen told the writer that she would have liked to make a tree that looked "more natural." Although she thought that a naturalistic depiction could have been achieved by adding details such as bark, twigs, and leaves, Karen stated that her omission of these elements could be attributed to the belief that she would not be able to draw them correctly.

Karen drew a very large tree that was formed using one continuous line. The drawing and her immediate response to it leads the writer to believe that Karen's effort was minimal and served only to comply with the request (Hammer, 1980). However, when looking at the drawing in greater depth, it appears that the simplicity and size of Karen's response could signify impulsivity or aggressive tendencies (Oster & Crone, 2004). Even though Karen's

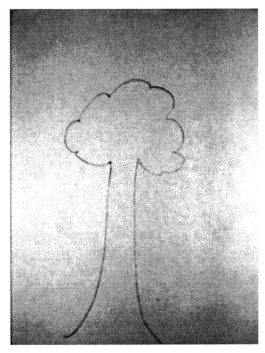

Figure 7.14. Karen's HTP Achromatic Tree.

demeanor contradicted a trait of aggression, some underlying aggressive tendencies may still be present; which could likely be related to the argumentative relationship she had with her mother. Just as it was absent in her house response, there is also no groundline present in Karen's tree drawing. When considered together with the lack of a root system, this may once more raise questions concerning her stability and vulnerability to stress.

The image of a tree can allow for the expression of unconscious, longstanding, and sometimes negative feelings toward the self, because it is less "close to home" than the house (home life) or person (more conscious view of self; Hammer, 1980). In this case, Karen's faintly drawn, simplistic tree might convey not only a lack of confidence in her artistic ability, but also a poor self-concept, lack of "ego-strength," feelings of inadequacy, or potential fear of seeking satisfaction from the environment (Hammer, 1980).

Achromatic Person

Karen's achromatic person response was preceded by a directive from the writer that she "try her best not to use a stick-figure." The pre-assessment interview revealed that Karen had little confidence in her artistic abilities

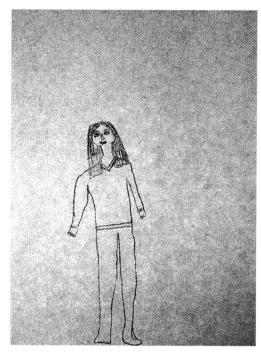

Figure 7.15. Karen's HTP Achromatic Person.

(especially in the area of drawing), and that she preferred to employ the use of stick-figures when drawing people. She began to work by creating an outline of the entire figure, from head to shirt, and then added pants and feet. Hands were depicted next and appeared quite small, with almost indiscernible fingers. Details such as eyes, lashes, brows, a nose and mouth were added next, followed lastly by hair.

Karen informed the writer that this person was her younger sister, Kelly. It has been shown that while the drawing of a person may often be a depiction of a significant other, it may also be an object upon which the subject's own personality traits are projected (Hammer, 1980). To that extent, the short arms, tiny hands, and rigidity of the figure may represent Karen's own need for control over her emotions or contacts with the environment (Hammer, 1980). The legs and body of Karen's person are quite long, and may suggest a striving for autonomy. At the same time, the tiny, diametrically opposed feet suggest instability and dependency (Oster & Crone, 2004). Light but excessive shading of the figure's hair may reflect underlying anxiety, and the visibility of the shoulders through the hair could be a sign of Karen's immaturity. Moreover, the groundline has yet again been omitted and the figure is leaning slightly; these factors might indicate instability or a need for support (Oster & Crone, 2004). Karen's potential instability could also be reflected in the unevenness of the shoulders and arms of the figure (Hammer, 1980).

Chromatic House-Tree-Person

The chromatic HTP series immediately followed the discussion of Karen's achromatic person response. It has been shown that conducting a second series with color (which can lead to effect), when emotional arousal is potentially high, may help reveal deeper, unconscious layers of a subject's personality (Hammer, 1980).

House

Karen was given the directive, "Now, draw a house in crayon," and responded by choosing blue to draw the entire outline of a house. She added a front door and windows before coloring in the house with blue. Brown was used next to color in the roof, followed by black to draw the doorknob and garage door windows. Karen drew the house from the same perspective seen in her achromatic response, and depicted almost identical features, including a large front window, a small front door, and a garage door with tiny windows. During the discussion, Karen informed the writer that the houses were indeed the same and represented the blue house that was her first home with her mother and stepfather.

Karen showed improved planning ability in this response, as this time she was able to fit the entire house within the drawing page. However, as was illustrated in the achromatic response, there was no depiction of a ground-line or inclusion of a chimney, which once again reflected the potential lack of stability and warmth within the home environment. Karen's second house has fewer windows than in the achromatic response and are shown completely bare, while the front door is no longer shown on the baseline of the house. These elements once again raise questions about accessibility to the house, in addition to Karen's personality, as well as potential ambiguity about, or desired control of, contacts with the environment (Hammer, 1980).

Personality clues hinted at in the achromatic series are often more clear-cut in the chromatic drawings (Hammer, 1980). Therefore, improvements in the depiction of certain key elements in the chromatic response may suggest a more positive prognosis. Apart from improved planning in the drawing's execution, the features of Karen's chromatic house drawing show little improvement; the front door is less accessible, there are fewer windows to provide access to the surrounding environment, and the home still appears to be unstable. The colors might also suggest a need to control behavior or inhibit emotional expression (blue), or signify repression (brown and black),

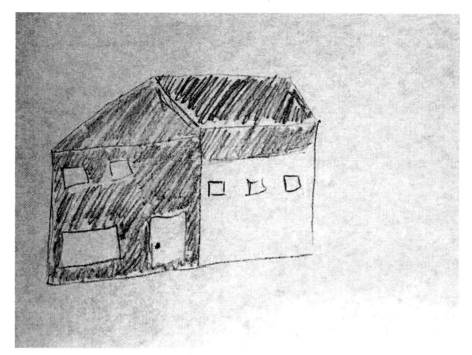

Figure 7.16. Karen's HTP Chromatic House. (For color version, see Plate 21, p. 119.)

despite Karen's statement about the house as representing one from her past (Hammer, 1980). The house seems likely then to be a representation of Karen's experience of an unstable family environment, as well as an expression of her need for warmth and support from her family (especially her mother), in the development of a stronger self-concept and self-worth.

Tree

In the chromatic tree response, the writer clearly saw Karen expend a greater effort on the task and observed an increase in the time spent on the picture in comparison to the achromatic response. Karen began by using a brown crayon to draw and fill in the trunk, and then she drew and colored in the crown of the tree with green. This tree was almost identical to the achromatic version, except that it was a little smaller, possibly because Karen oriented the paper horizontally this time. The lines of the crown and trunk were drawn faintly, and colored in lightly and evenly. Similar to the achromatic response, Karen's light depiction of the tree may represent insecurity, and instability is suggested by the absence of a groundline (Oster & Crone, 2004). Karen gave no indication of a root structure, which reinforces her potential need for more stability and support. There is also an apparent lack

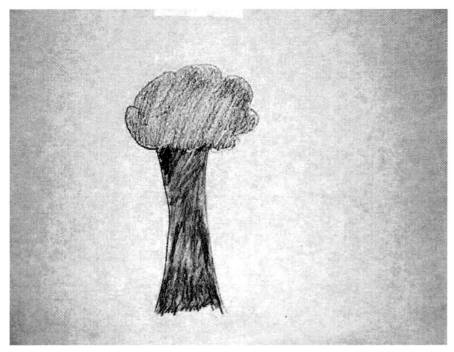

Figure 7.17. Karen's HTP Chromatic Tree. (For color version, see Plate 22, p. 119.)

of a branch system, which may reflect Karen's potential need for control when making contacts within her environment. Further, despite the tree's naturalistic depiction of color, the colors chosen could once again indicate a need for control (green) and repression of emotions (brown) (Hammer, 1980).

Person

The final task for Karen was the chromatic person. Karen started the drawing by using purple to draw a shirt, upon which she wrote the letters "LTD," before coloring it in. Karen informed the writer that these letters stood for a clothing line sold in the store at which she is employed. Black was then used to outline the head, draw the nose, eyes and mouth of the figure. Karen then took care in adding details to the face, as she applied yellow to depict long hair, red for large lips and green for the iris of each eye. Blue was then used to create the pants and feet of the person; Karen colored the pants with blue and the shoes with black.

Karen identified this figure to be her sister, Kelly, who was also the subject of her achromatic response. Karen's choice of subject is no surprise to the writer, considering the high possibility that she may still harbor feelings

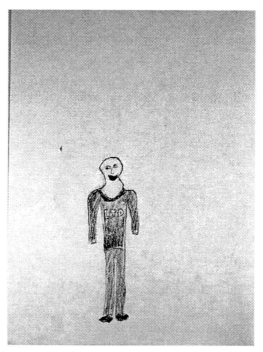

Figure 7.18. Karen's HTP Chromatic Person. (For color version, see Plate 23, p. 120.)

of resentment toward Kelly for taking her "role" in the family. By depicting Kelly, Karen could have been trying to shift the focus to someone other than herself, in an attempt to exert control over her emotional expression. It is likely that this picture is not simply a portrait of Kelly, but rather a projection of Karen's own personality traits.

Karen's drawn figure still appears to be quite small in size when compared to the space of the drawing page, which might parallel her own perceived insignificance in her family and communicate potential feelings of inadequacy (Hammer, 1980). There is an emphasis on the large, red mouth, which may be a sign of immaturity or oral aggression. Most remarkable in the chromatic response may be the omission of the hands. This oversight could reflect a lack of control or feelings of inadequacy (Oster & Crone, 2004).

Recommendations and Conclusion

Karen's responses to both the achromatic and chromatic HTP assessments may reflect deep-seated feelings about the impact that her experience of an unstable family environment has had on her self-concept and confidence. Her drawings may also suggest that the perceived lack of support from her family (especially her mother) has led Karen to find it necessary to inhibit the expression of her emotions and control her interactions with the environment. The writer recommends that Karen consider engaging in art therapy on a regular basis, so that she may further explore her feelings about her family, find a constructive outlet for emotional expression, as well as develop increased confidence and a stronger self-concept.

Conclusion and Recommendations

The results of Karen's KFD response (not included in this book), when taken in conjunction with her psychosocial history and the responses to the HTP and CATA (not included in this book) assessments may indicate that Karen desires more warmth, stability and support from her family. Karen's KFD response (not included in this book) may have been an attempt to create a picture of a family with these desired characteristics. However, the elements of the drawing suggest that Karen may be dealing with underlying feelings of inadequacy, dependency, and isolation, in regard to her family situation and relationship with her mother.

Individual art therapy is recommended so that Karen may learn how to express her needs, gain more self-confidence and build up her self-esteem. Eventually inviting Karen's family, especially her mother and sister, into the art therapy sessions would be a positive way to get clarification about the feelings of resentment, rejection, and inadequacy Karen may feel has affected her relationship with her mother since Kelly was born.

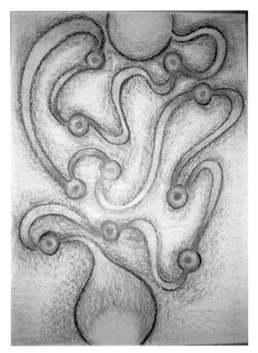

Plate 1. (Figure 2.1. Sandy's ATDA Response.)

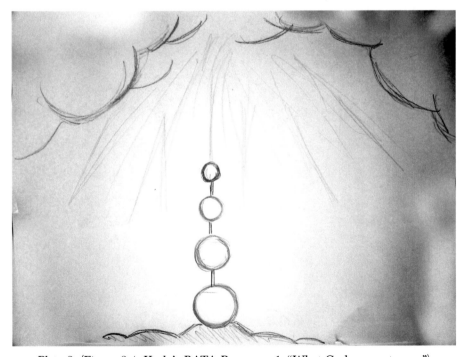

Plate 2. (Figure 3.4. Karla's BATA Response 1, "What God means to me.")

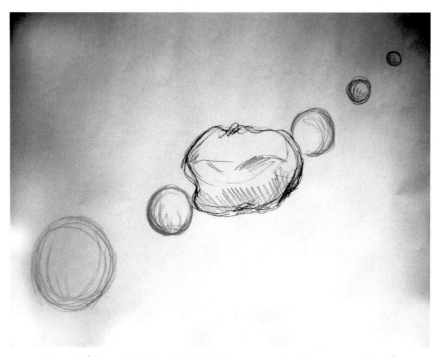

Plate 3. (Figure 3.5. Karla's BATA Response 2 – Opposite of God.)

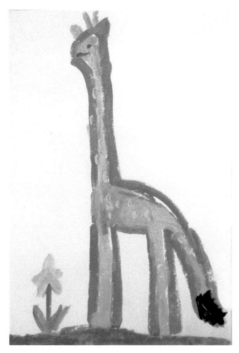

Plate 4. (Figure 5.1. S's CATA Paint Response.)

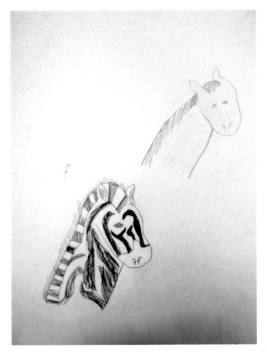

Plate 5. (Figure 5.3. S's CATA Drawing Response.)

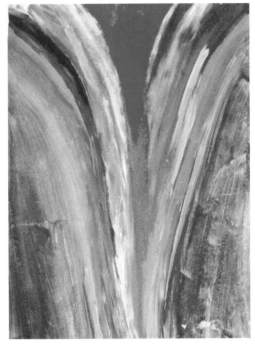

Plate 6. (Figure 5.6. Lucy's CATA Paint Response.)

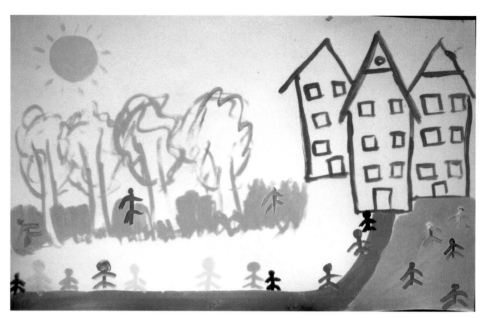

Plate 7. (Figure 5.7. D's CATA Paint Response.)

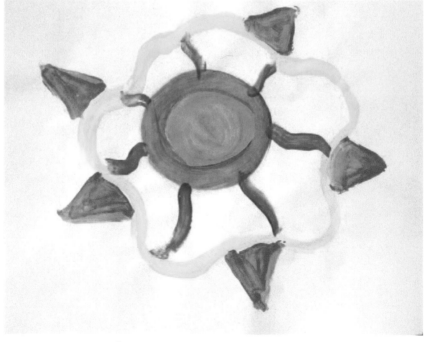

Plate 8. (Figure 5.11. Sandy's CATA Paint Response.)

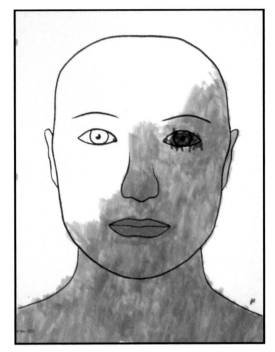

Plate 9. (Figure 6.1. Pam's SDT Picture 1 Response.)

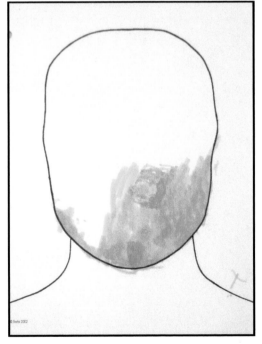

Plate 10. (Figure 6.2. Pam's SDT Picture 2 Response.)

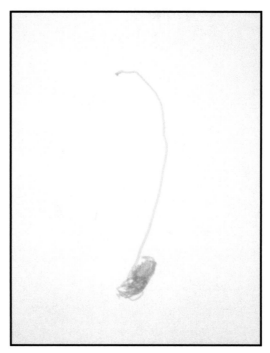

Plate 11. (Figure 6.3. Pam's SDT Picture 3 Response.)

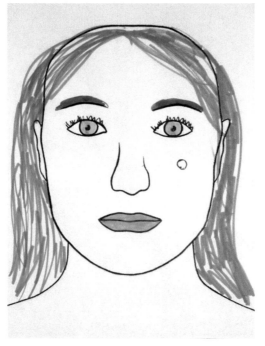

Plate 12. (Figure 6.4. Sandy's SDT Picture 1 Response.)

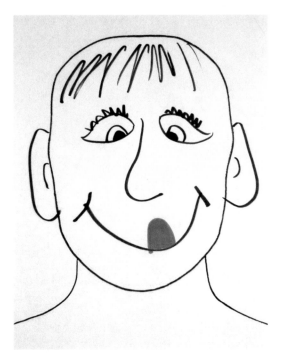

Plate 13. (Figure 6.5. Sandy's SDT Picture 2 Response.)

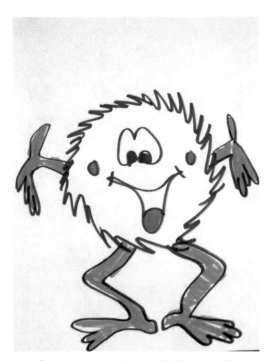

Plate 14. (Figure 6.6. Sandy's SDT Picture 3 Response.)

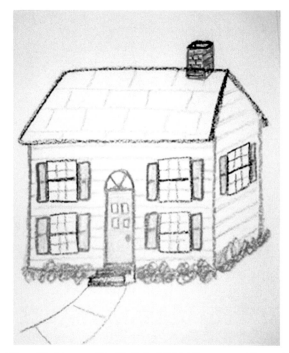

Plate 15. (Figure 7.2. Holly's HTP Chromatic House.)

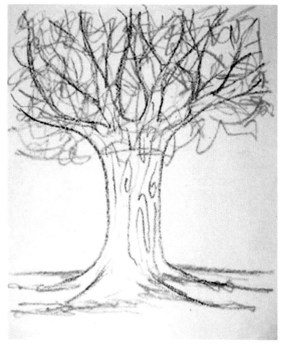

Plate 16. (Figure 7.4. Holly's HTP Chromatic Tree.)

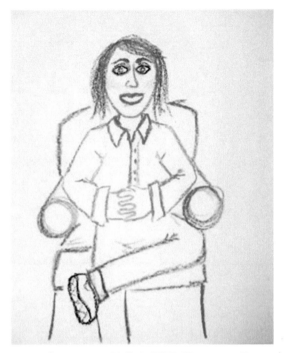

Plate 17. (Figure 7.6. Holly's HTP Chromatic Person.)

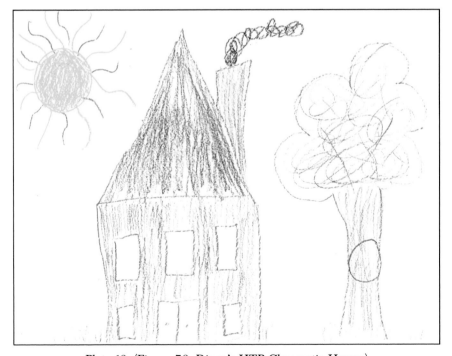

Plate 18. (Figure 7.8. Diane's HTP Chromatic House.)

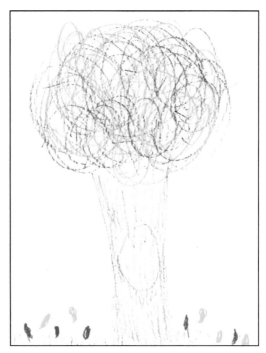

Plate 19. (Figure 7.10. Diane's HTP Chromatic Tree.)

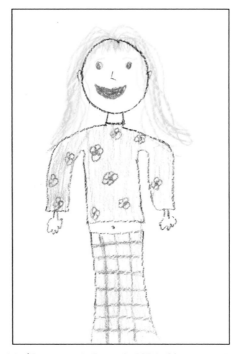

Plate 20. (Figure 7.12. Diane's HTP Chromatic Person.)

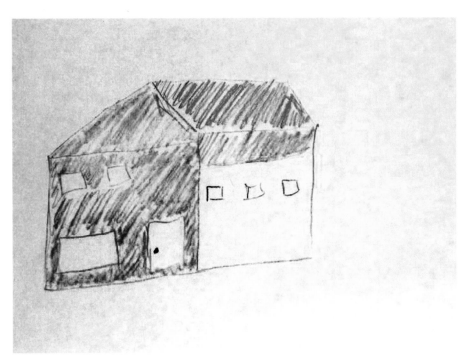

Plate 21. (Figure 7.16. Karen's HTP Chromatic House.)

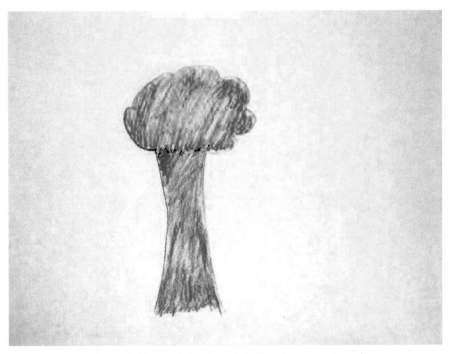

Plate 22. (Figure 7.17. Karen's HTP Chromatic Tree.)

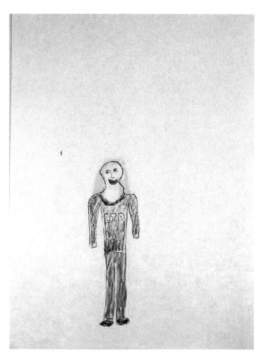

Plate 23. (Figure 7.18. Karen's HTP Chromatic Person.)

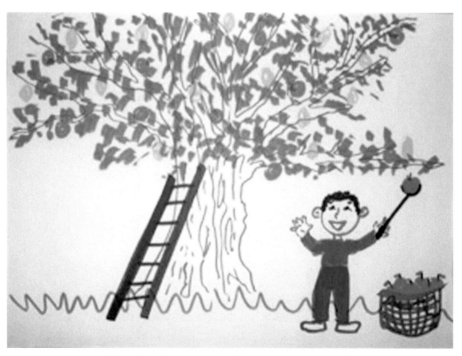

Plate 24. (Figure 9.1. Holly's PPAT Response.)

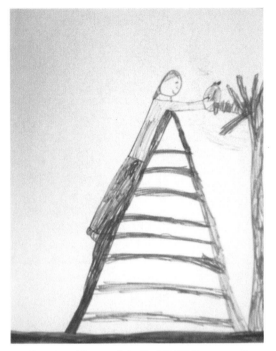

Plate 25. (Figure 9.2. S's PPAT Response.)

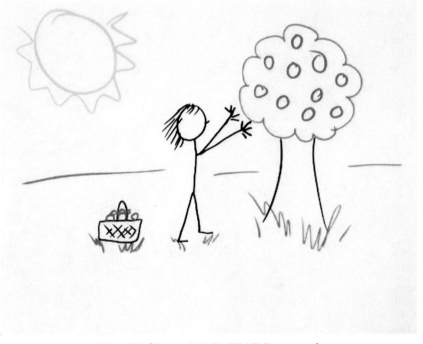

Plate 26. (Figure 9.5. L's PPAT Response.)

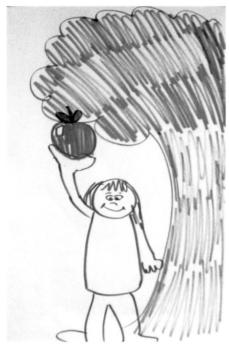

Plate 27. (Figure 9.8. Sandy's PPAT Response.)

Plate 28. (Figure 11.2. Alexander's CATA Paint Response.)

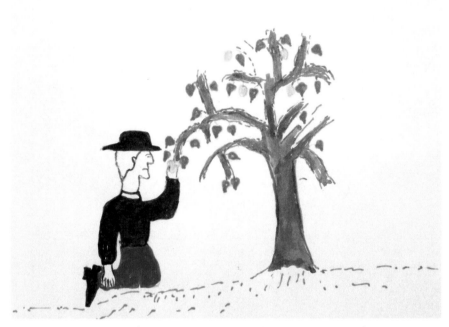

Plate 29. (Figure 11.11. Alexander's PPAT Response.)

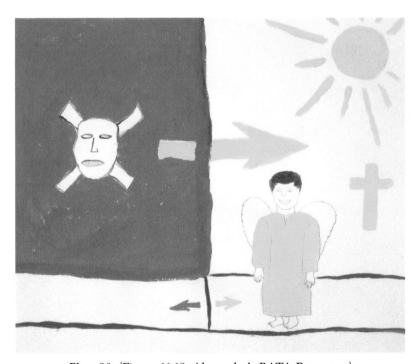

Plate 30. (Figure 11.12. Alexander's BATA Response.)

Chapter 8

KINETIC FAMILY DRAWING
ASSESSMENT (KFD)

The earliest literature recordings found on family drawings was the Draw-A-Family (D-A-F) test (Hulse, 1951, 1952). While Hammer (1980), Koppitz (1968), and DiLeo (1970) went on to describe the use of the D-A-F in their comprehensive texts, it wasn't until Burns & Kaufman (1970) that children were asked to draw their families *doing something*. (The operative point here is the concept of asking the drawer to imagine him or her self in a family drawing *doing something*.) It was thought that the requirement to add movement to the akinetic drawing would stimulate a child's feelings as related to the self concept, intra-familial, and interpersonal relationships. As a clinician for over 30 years, Horovitz (2002, 2005, 2007) has found the KFD to be the single most important projective tool in her arsenal. This simple projective task can elicit information that recreates all the transitional conflicts handed down from generation-to-generation (as gleaned from the IP genogram).

While analysis of the KFD symbols are expressed in great detail in Burns & Kaufman's opus, the authors again point the reader back to that book in order to offer the reader a more detailed account of the symbolic meanings of barriers, competition, action items, compartmentalization, and so on.

However, regarding the administration of the KFD, Burns & Kaufman (1972) suggest the following administration (p. 5):

> A sheet of plain white, 8 1/2 x 11 inch paper is placed on the table directly in front of the (drawer). A No. 2 pencil is placed in the center of the paper and the (subject) is asked to "Draw a picture of everyone in your family doing something, including you, *DOING* something. Try to draw whole people, not cartoons or stick people. Remember, make everyone *DOING* something – some kind of action."

125

Now it is the next action that the authors recommend against. It is stated that the examiner leave the room, leaving the subject unaccompanied. Under no conditions would the authors recommend this, both from a liability stand-point as well as that of clinical examiner. One cannot possibly interpret the drawing without watching who was drawn first, glean erasures and their sub-sequent projective meaning, and so forth. As well, when working with an emotionally challenged population, leaving the room would be considered ethically negligent.

Finally, Horovitz has instructed her students for years to create a graph-like grid, which could be found at local office supply stores, scanned into a computer and printed out on acetate so that this "grid" structure can be thrown over the KFD response. By doing this, one can measure the exact proximity and/or distance between family members or environmental images produced in the subtest. This offers the clinician further information into the environmental familial-triggers of the subject.

As well, an analysis sheet can be found at the end of this chapter, again offering the administrant another way of mapping such items as actions between figure, symbols, erasures, omission of figures, and so on.

Identified Patient: Nathan

CA: 26.9

DOB: April 5, 1979

Testing Date: April 2, 2006

Administrant: Sarah L. Eksten

Assessments Administered: ATDA, KFD, SDT

See Chapters 1, 2, and 10 for further examples regarding Nathan.

Refer to Appendix A for Genogram, Timeline, Behavioral Observations, and Psychosocial Indicators.

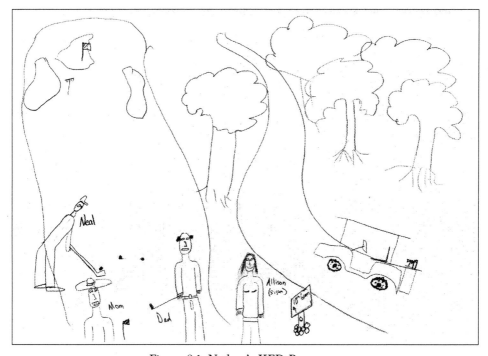

Figure 8.1. Nathan's KFD Response.

The individuals in the picture, from left to right, were identified as himself, his mother (Jane), his father (Charlie), and sister (Allison). They were on a golf course, Mt. Pleasant, near Baltimore, MD. While drawing the individuals, he commented on his inability to draw people. The administrant asked him if his family were conversing, what they would be talking about. He said that if his family engaged in a conversation they would be fighting about golf (i.e., whose ball was whose; which was closer; whether to re-hit a ball; etc.). This would then turn into fighting about anything. Nathan said that this fighting, though, only occurred while they were golfing. He said he thought it was because golf was a stressful game and it built up aggression in all of them. Nathan said his sister would not play and would just stand by the sidelines to watch. He said that she usually does her own thing all the time and, for the most part, does not participate in family outings.

If one examines the picture closer, it can be seen that the golf course only encapsulated both the parents and part of Nathan. This could re-emphasize the fact that the sister does not participate in many family functions. It could also indicate that she may be ostracized from the family. Looking at the individuals in his picture, Nathan drew himself as transparent, with the ability to see the continuation of the golf course, suggesting some immaturity and/or regression connected to both the competition and family of origin issues (Oster & Crone, 2004). The drawing of himself also lacked hands, possibly signifying feelings of trouble or inadequacy (Oster & Crone, 2004). In addition, his figure was drawn as a profile, perhaps indicating evasiveness, possible paranoia, or feeling excessively withdrawn (Oster & Crone, 2004). He displayed his mother as having a large mouth, emphasizing her teeth. This may connote that Nathan views his mother as being orally aggressive or sarcastic (Oster & Crone, 2004). He also pointed out the small breasts on his sister, and the lack of them on his mother. This may indicate a sexualization of his sister, but not toward his mother. To further emphasize the de-sexualization of his mother, he only portrayed her from the waist up, completely eliminating any body parts from below the waist. Nathan also noted that the zipper of his father's pants looked like a penis. According to Freud's psychosexual stages, Nathan may still be caught in the Phallic Stage, identifying with his father and becoming as much like him as possible in order to gain his mother's love. The wheels on the golf cart were reinforced, possibly signifying some anxiety or aggression (Oster & Crone, 2004). Some of the trees were drawn faintly, which could suggest feelings of inadequacy or indecisiveness (Oster & Crone, 2004). Two of the trees had two lines for a trunk and a looped crown, which could display impulsive characteristics (Oster & Crone, 2004). There were some roots at the bases of the trees; however, they were minimal, which may insinuate that Nathan may repress some of his emotions (Oster & Crone, 2004). Also, no definite groundline was present, which could imply that Nathan is vulnerable to stress (Oster & Crone, 2004). Also of interest is that all the family members (with the exception of Nathan) are facing the viewer and are thus turned away from Nathan and his impending shot. This might also reflect his feeling shunned and ignored by his nuclear family members.

Recommendations and Conclusions

By comparing all three assessments, overall conclusions can be determined regarding Nathan's characteristics. The fact that Nathan used pencil for all drawings, even when he was able to use coloring media, may conclude that Nathan is afraid to explore any emotions surrounding the drawings he completed since color is known to extract feelings and emotions. In addition, all the drawings, for the most part, lacked symmetry, indicating that Nathan may have inadequate feelings of security in his emotional life (Hammer, 1958). This challenges the score Nathan obtained in the Stimulus Drawing (see Chapter 10) that indicated he may be aware of his emotions and can freely express them through art. All the drawings contained straightline strokes, which may be present in individuals who tend to be assertive (Hammer, 1958). The drawings of himself in each picture lacked hands, possibly signifying feelings of trouble or inadequacy (Oster & Crone, 2004). In the drawings that contained trees, most of them had two lines for a trunk and a looped crown, possibly displaying impulsive characteristics (Oster & Crone, 2004). All the trees in the pictures either had no or a very minimal root system, which may insinuate that Nathan represses some of his emotions (Oster & Crone, 2004). Each picture was lacking a definite groundline, which could imply that Nathan is vulnerable to stress or that he is unstable (Oster & Crone, 2004). Both the ATDA (see Chapter 2) and SDT (see Chapter 10) uncovered possible unconscious thoughts of escape from some situation in his life.

From reviewing the drawings, the writer concluded that Nathan falls between Lowenfeld and Brittain's Schematic Stage (7–9 years) and Gang Age (9–12 years) (Horovitz, 2002). The drawings were more conceptual rather than perceptual. They also had a bold, direct representation with the organization of objects being mostly two-dimensional and there being little overlap; however, there was some awareness to detail. In addition, Nathan expressed the self-consciousness of his drawings. There still seemed to be no understanding of shade and shadow; although, there was less exaggeration of body parts and more stiffness of figures.

The administrant suggests that although there seemed to be no significant indications of problems that were a cause for concern from reviewing these three assessments, she feels that Nathan may still benefit from occasional Art Therapy to release any stress he may be encountering. It may also be beneficial in that it may help him become more in touch with his feelings and emotions, and he may learn ways of expressing them. Art Therapy can also be used as an opportunity to sort out any feelings of trouble or inadequacy that may be occurring, or to explore his impulsivity.

K-F-D ANALYSIS SHEET

Name: _____ Nathan _____ Age: **26.9** Date of Birth: **04/02/1979** Sex: **M**

I. STYLE(S) (Circle)
    A. Compartmentalization
    B. Edging
    C. Encapsulation
    D. Folded Compartmentalization
    E. Lining on the Bottom
    F. Lining on the Top
    G. Underling individual figures

II. SYMBOL(S)
    A. Barriers (course line) D. _____
    B. _____ E. _____
    C. _____ F. _____

III. (A) ACTIONS OF INDIVIDUAL FIGURES

Figure	Action
1. Self	Golfing
2. Mother	Standing
3. Father	Standing
4. Older Brother	N/A
5. Older Sister	N/A
6. Younger Brother	N/A
7. Younger Sister	Standing
8. Other (Specify)	N/A

(B) ACTIONS BETWEEN INDIVIDUAL FIGURES

Figure	Action	Recipient
1. Self	N/A	
2. Mother	N/A	
3. Father	N/A	
4. O.B.	N/A	
5. O.S.	N/A	
6. Y.B.	N/A	
7. Y.S.	N/A	
8. Other	N/A	

IV. CHARACTERISTICS OF K-F-D FIGURES

A. Arm Extensions
  1. Self   5. O.S.
  2. Mother 6. Y.B.
  3. Father 7. Y.S.
  4. O.B.   8. Other

B. Elevated Figures
  1. Self   5. O.S.
  2. Mother 6. Y.B.
  3. Father 7. Y.S.
  4. O.B.   8. Other

C. Erasures N/A
  1. Self   5. O.S.
  2. Mother 6. Y.B.
  3. Father 7. Y.S.
  4. O.B.   8. Other

D. Figures on Back N/A
  1. Self   5. O.S.
  2. Mother 6. Y.B.
  3. Father 7. Y.S.

E. Hanging N/A
  1. Self   5. O.S.
  2. Mother 6. Y.B.
  3. Father 7. Y.S.
  4. O.B.   8. Other

B. Location of Self
  Bottom Left

C. Distance of Self From:
Mother .25" Brother _____
Father 2.75" Sister 4.25"
Other (Specify) _____

F. Omission of Body Parts
  1. Self   5. O.S.
  2. Mother 6. Y.B.
  3. Father 7. Y.S.
  4. O.B.   8. Other

G. Omission of Figures N/A
  1. Self   5. O.S.
  2. Mother 6. Y.B.
  3. Father 7. Y.S.
  4. O.B.   8. Other

H. Picasso Eyes N/A
  1. Self   5. O.S.
  2. Mother 6. Y.B.
  3. Father 7. Y.S.
  4. O.B.   8. Other

I. Rotated Figures N/A
  1. Self   5. O.S.
  2. Mother 6. Y.B.
  3. Father 7. Y.S.
  4. O.B.   8. Other

V. K-F-D Grid
A. Height
  1. Self 2.25" 5. O.S.
  2. M. 1.5"   6. Y.B.
  3. F. 2.75" 7. Y.S. 2.25"
  4. O.B. _____ 8. Other _____

Figure 8.2. Nathan's KFD Analysis Sheet.

Identified Patient: Adam

CA: 24.8

DOB: March 13, 1986

Administrant: Jordan M. Kroll

Test Date: November 19, 2006

Assessment Administered: KFD

Refer to Appendix A for Genogram, Timeline, Behavioral Observations, and Psychosocial Indicators.

Behavioral Observations

With defense mechanisms flying high, Adam began by drawing two circles, a triangle, a square, and a parallelogram, each replete with dashes for eyes and mouth, and a small cross rooted underneath as a body. This response to the KFD directive was not overly conducive as an art therapy assessment, and he was encouraged to start anew. He then produced a drawing which, while it would still be assessed at Lowenfeld and Brittain's Schematic Stage (7–9 years), offered much more in the way of insightful content.

Five stick figures arranged in an "X" shape represent mother and father at the top, middle brother in the middle of the page, and Adam in the lower right corner. This large X is mirrored by the smaller X's of the bodies, a crucifix, and a window, and may suggest conflict and a desire to control it (Burns & Kaufman, 1972). The figures are compartmentalized with light, subtle lines between each of them, and frame-like corners are drawn to fill up the entire page. These barriers are common in social isolates (Burns & Kaufman, 1972) and true to Adam's situation. He moved to Michigan with his girlfriend, and feels he has not established strong social ties for himself apart from her family and friends.

Susan, Adam's mother, is located in the top-left and is the largest figure. This "Visual Giver of Love" showers hearts on the family – a positive transfer of energy (Burns & Kaufman, 1972, pp. 36–43). In the drawing, Adam is the furthest away from this "love." Lee (father) is the upper right figure and a "Humble Grower of Life." He is turned from the viewer and attending a small plant. Lee is a retired Soil Conservation Scientist and an avid gardener. Adam recognized a positive influence from his father throughout his life. Perhaps Adam is now feeling like a plant that needs a little watering. Hudson, the oldest child at 30 and a youth pastor in Florida, lies in the lower left at the foot of a cross. The rotation of his figure makes it look as though he is

falling down, as he stares wide-eyed at the viewer. Adam let on that his relationship to Hudson was not as close as to his other brother, Michael. Adam
places Michael in the center of the page in a somewhat precarious position
atop a globe. He is "Effectively Wandering the World," and his elevated status may tell of Adam seeing him as the dominant sibling (Burns & Kaufman,
1972, p. 18), though this idea is contested by the fact that he is the smallest
figure and by Adam saying that he would have placed the brothers in a row
had the space allowed. The tension exhibited in both Hudson's and
Michael's proximity possibly alludes to Adam's envy of their direction in life.
Hudson and his wife were recently blessed with a daughter, making Adam
an uncle, and Michael is attending graduate school. Finally, Adam sees himself as "Curiously Searching the Possibilities." His back is to the viewer as he
gazes out of a nondescript window. One gets the feeling that he is waiting for
something – perhaps the water (nurturance) that he is not currently receiving, or simply a new chapter to write or quest to conquer.

That all of the figures are stick people is seen by Burns and Kaufman
(1972) as a defense mechanism, and the omission of hands and feet suggests
a denial of function and possibly helplessness. All of the heads, especially
those of the parents, are rather large and may illustrate a preoccupation with
intellectual pursuits and/or wisdom that Adam's family system holds in high
regard. The eyes are also oversized, possibly representing "vision" in life.
Adam, who in the drawing has no eyes, is apparently lacking or incomplete
in his vision at this point. A final element in the drawing is the word "ONE"
at top center. Adam opined that U2's song "One" may be the best modern
song ever written, and including this as a title in his drawing shows a hope
in the strength and love of a family unit to overcome all possible tension,
conflict, and uncertainty in life.

Conclusion

What Adam's KFD assessment sacrifices concerning domestic issues as
well as cognitive and artistic development, it makes up for in uniqueness of
execution and in existential material. His guarded approach and attempt to
not take this event very seriously reveal Adam's dualistic view of life's experiences. On one hand are the things he considers important and worth every
effort in which to achieve success, and on the other, everything else that is
expendable, trivial, even silly. We are also confronted with a rather timely
still-frame of a young man's journey through life, and the respective place of
his family members in this.

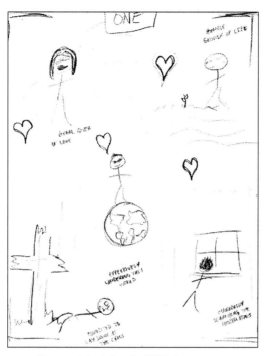

Figure 8.3. Adam's KFD Response.

K-F-D ANALYSIS SHEET

Name: ADAM   Age: 24   Date of Birth: 3/13/82   Sex: Male

I. STYLE(S) (Circle)
- Ⓐ Compartmentalization
- Ⓑ Edging
- C. Encapsulation
- D. Folded Compartmentalization
- E. Lining on the Bottom
- F. Lining on the Top
- Ⓖ Underlining individual figures

II. SYMBOL(S)
- A. "ONE"   D.
- B. Hearts   E.
- C. Cross   F.

III. (A) ACTIONS OF INDIVIDUAL FIGURES

Figure	Action
1. Self	Searching (looking)
2. Mother	Giving Love
3. Father	Growing /slanting
4. Older Brother	Religious submission
5. Older Sister	
6. Younger Brother	
7. Younger Sister	
8. Other (Specify) Older Brother	Wandering

(B) ACTIONS BETWEEN INDIVIDUAL FIGURES

Figure	Action	Recipient
1. Self		
2. Mother	Showering Love	All
3. Father		
4. O.B.		
5. O.S.		
6. Y.B.		
7. Y.S.		
8. Other		

IV. CHARACTERISTICS OF K-F-D FIGURES

A. Arm Extensions
1. Self	5. O.S.
2. Mother	6. Y.B.
3. Father	7. Y.S.
4. O.B.	8. Other

B. Elevated Figures
1 Self	5. O.S.
② Mother	6. Y.B.
③ Father	7. Y.S.
④ O.B.	8. Other

C. Erasures
1. Self	5. O.S.
2. Mother	6. Y.B.
3. Father	7. Y.S.
4. O.B.	8. Other

D. Figures on Back
1. Self	5. O.S.
2. Mother	6. Y.B.
3. Father	7. Y.S.

E. Hanging
1. Self	5. O.S.
2. Mother	6. Y.B.
3. Father	7. Y.S.
4. O.B.	8. Other

B. Location of Self
Bottom - right

C. Distance of Self From:
Mother 18 cm   Brother 6 cm
Father 12 cm   Sister X
Other (Specify) OB - 7 cm

F. Omission of Body Parts
① Self	5. O.S.
② Mother	6. Y.B.
③ Father	7. Y.S.
④ O.B.	⑧ Other O.B.

G. Omission of Figures
1. Self	5. O.S.
2. Mother	6. Y.B.
3. Father	7. Y.S.
4. O.B.	8. Other

H. Picasso Eyes
1. Self	5. O.S.
② Mother	6. Y.B.
3. Father	7. Y.S.
4. O.B.	8. Other

I. Rotated Figures
1. Self	5. O.S.
2. Mother	6. Y.B.
3. Father	7. Y.S.
④ O.B.	8. Other

V. K-F-D Grid
A. Height
1. Self 5 cm S.O.S.
2. M. 7 cm 6. Y.B.
3. F. 5 cm 7. Y.S.
4. O.B. 6 cm 8. Other 4.5 cm OB

Figure 8.4. Adam's KFD Analysis Sheet.

Identified Patient: D

DOB: May 27, 1986

CA: 22

Testing Dates: September 28, 2007

Administrant: M. Trinidad Selman P.

Assessments Administered: CATA, KFD

See Chapter 5 for a further example regarding D.

Refer to Appendix A for Genogram, Timeline, Behavioral Observations, and Psychosocial Indicators.

This is the third assessment D completed, hence she demonstrated very cooperative behavior and appeared less anxious than the last time we met for the HTP assessment (not included in this book). However, she asked if someone made a comment regarding her other drawings made during the CATA (see Chapter 5) and HTP (not included in this book) assessments, possibly indicating that she is concerned about the results of the drawing. D took approximately 15 minutes to draw the KFD, without talking and only erasing a few times. Upon completion, D talked about the scene she drew.

Figure 8.5. D's KFD Response.

Assessment Results

D described the above scene as a family ceremony held in her home country each year in October. In this ceremony, parents have to put a "Tika" in the forehead of their daughters and sons as a sign of blessing. The drawing represents the moment in which her father is putting a Tika in her forehead in the presence of her mother and brother.

The drawing is lacking a baseline and all the characters are floating in the middle of the page. Oster and Crone (2004) suggest that the lack of groundline in the tree drawing may indicate vulnerability to stress. The administrant noted that the order in which she drew the family was father (left), herself, mother (between her and her father), and brother at last (right, at the center of the page). The size of the brother's character is larger than the rest and is separated from the main scene. (As well, the brother is turned away from the ceremonial aspect of this event and instead faces the viewer rather than the family members, suggesting some sort of displacement from the family and possible estrangement.) When D was asked about what he was doing, she stated "he is just watching." Hammer (1980) suggests that the variation of the size in the members of the family may indicate the dominance and importance of each member for the individual.

The pressure and lines vary between the three figures at the left (father, mother, D) and the figure at the right (brother). Hammer (1980) stated that variations in pressure correspond to individuals who are perhaps more flexible and adaptable. The same author suggests that a continuous line frequently reinforced, is an indicative of anxiety and insecurity (Hammer, 1980). The excessive pressure also may indicate aggression (Burns & Kaufman, 1972). Oster and Crone (2004) state that heavy lines may elicit a sense of tension. D drew each figure with short, sketchy strokes, which is associated with anxiety and uncertainty (Hammer, 1980). The figures are drawn at the left of the midpoint of the page, which may suggest that the subject behave impulsively and seek immediate emotional satisfaction of needs and drives (Hammer, 1980). The author also pointed out that an individual who draws below the midpoint of the page, might feel insecure and inadequate and that this feeling is cause of depression of mood. In addition, the subject finds him/herself "reality-bound, oriented toward the concrete" (Hammer, 1980, p. 70). In general, the drawing has a lack of details, which suggests withdrawal tendencies, feelings of emptiness and reduced energy, characteristic of subjects with depression (Hammer, 1980).

The father is drawn from a side view perspective. The drawing of a person's profile may indicate evasiveness, a paranoid tendency, and withdrawn conduct (Oster & Crone, 2004). In the action of putting the "Tika" in D's forehead, he is drawn with a very long arm. This may suggest that he is controlling the environment (Burns & Kaufman, 1972) as well as an ambition or reaching out towards others (Oster & Crone, 2004). D's character position is very stiff. Moreover, her character is depicted with no hands. On one hand, Oster and Crone (2004) state that omitted arms may suggest inadequacy and helplessness, and no hands is an indicator of trouble and feelings of inadequacy. On the other hand, Burns and Kaufman (1972) suggest that the individual may have a conflict with the omitted part or denial of function. The mother's character is the only one shaded. Both, Burns and Kaufman (1972) and Oster and Crone (2004) suggest that shading in a drawing may indicate preoccupation, fixation or anxiety. When compared to the rest of the figures, she has short arms (only one is visible), which may indicate a tendency toward withdrawal, turning inward and inhibiting impulses (Oster & Crone, 2004). With regard to her brother's character, he is separated from the rest of the family members. Burns and Kaufman (1972) regard this situation of isolation as a form of compartmentalization. Although he is not in a box, he is still isolated from the rest of the family. The authors state "this style is typical of social isolates who try to cut off the feeling component between individual members of the family" (Burns & Kaufman, 1972). Both D and her brother have belts, which may suggest sexual conflicts or covert tension (Oster & Crone, 2004). The fact that D is close to her parents, leaving her brother aside, may indicate that she is trying to demonstrate increased status over her brother or to express feelings of acceptance or rejection (Oster & Crone, 2004). The same authors state "individuals who view themselves with a grater degree of significance in the family, compared to siblings, will often place themselves in closer proximity to the parents" (Oster & Crone, 2004, p. 64).

Discussion

D seemed more relaxed during this assessment than on the other assessments (CATA [see Chapter 5] and HTP [not included in this book]); however, the results of the KFD indicate that she became anxious with any artistic task. The drawing conveys a family interaction, where all the members are close together doing the same activity. Although the brother's character is a little isolated, he is still part of the ceremony. The physical closeness between the family members may indicate that they all have a close relationship and she is a "well-adjusted" girl (Burns & Kaufman, 1972).

Comparing the results of the three assessments (CATA [see Chapter 5], HTP [not included in this book], & KFD), the administrant can say that D is living a tough period away from her home country and family. Her artworks denote she feels insecure, anxious, and possibly with signs of depression. The administrant recommends that D seek for support as prevention of stress and a mood disorder (depression) so that she can be less worried and more peaceful during her college years.

K-F-D ANALYSIS SHEET

Name: D   Age: 21   Sex: F

I. STYLE (s)
- (A) Compartmentalization
- B. Edging
- C. Encapsulation
- D. Folded Compartmentalization
- E. Lining on the Bottom
- F. Lining on the Top
- G. Underlining individual figures

II. SYMBOL (s)

A. -	D. -
B. -	E. -
C. -	F. -

III. (A) ACTIONS OF INDIVIDUAL FIGURES

Figure	Action
1. Self	receiving
2. Mother	watching
3. Father	putting "tika"
4. Older brother	watching
5. Older sister	-
6. Younger brother	-
7. Younger sister	-
8. Other (Specify)	-

(B) ACTIONS BETWEEN INDIVIDUAL FIGURES

Figure	Action	Recipient
1. Self	receiving	dad
2. Mother	watching	D and father
3. Father	putting "tika"	D
4. Older brother	watching	family (and viewers)
5. Older sister	-	
6. Younger brother	-	
7. Younger sister	-	
8. Other (Specify)	-	

IV. CHARACTERISTICS OF INDIVIDUAL KFD FIGURES

A. Arm extensions
1. Self	5. O.S.	
(2) Mother	6. Y.B.	
(3) Father	7. Y.S.	
(4) O.B.	8. Other	

F. Omission of body parts
(1) Self	5. O.S.
2. Mother	6. Y.B.
3. Father	7. Y.S.
4. O.B.	8. Other

B. Elevated Figures
(1) Self	5. O.S.
(2) Mother	6. Y.B.
(3) Father	7. Y.S.
4. O.B.	8. Other

G. Omission of figures
1. Self	5. O.S.
2. Mother	6. Y.B.
3. Father	7. Y.S.
4. O.B.	8. Other

C. Erasures
(1) Self	5. O.S.
2. Mother	6. Y.B.
(3) Father	7. Y.S.
4. O.B.	8. Other

H. Picasso Eye
1. Self	5. O.S.
2. Mother	6. Y.B.
3. Father	7. Y.S.
4. O.B.	8. Other

D. Figures on back
1. Self	5. O.S.
2. Mother	6. Y.B.
3. Father	7. Y.S.
4. O.B.	8. Other

I. Rotated figures
1. Self	5. O.S.
2. Mother	6. Y.B.
3. Father	7. Y.S.
4. O.B.	8. Other

E. Hanging
1. Self	5. O.S.
2. Mother	6. Y.B.
3. Father	7. Y.S.
4. O.B.	8. Other

V. KFD GRID

A. Height
1. Self: 9cm.	5. O.S.:
2. M: 8cm.	6. Y.B.:
3. F: 8.5cm.	7. Y.S.:
4. O.B.: 12cm.	8. Other:

B. Location of self:
Between mother and O.B.

C. Distance of self from:
Mother: 0
Father: 0
Other (Specify): O.B. 1cm.

Figure 8.6. D's KFD Analysis Sheet.

Personal Comment

It was very useful to have administered the three assessments to the same person; I realized that the client's concerns were expressed in the three of them. By analyzing the output of these assessments, specifically the way they illustrate important issues of a person, I clearly see the value of performing art assessments.

Identified Patient: Elizabeth

DOB: 1977

CA: 30

Testing Date: November 16, 2007

Administrant: Rebecca Ward

Assessment Administered: KFD

Refer to Appendix A for Genogram, Timeline, Behavioral Observations, and Psychosocial Indicators.

Elizabeth began her drawing with the shape of the table and proceeded to draw each of her family members seated around the table. She began with her younger brother, Ben, and continued drawing clockwise around the table, ending with her father. The drawing is placed in the upper left-hand quadrant of the page, which may express an "obsessive compulsive system of emotional control" (Burns & Kaufman, 1972, p. 297). The drawing completely lacked any surrounding environment as well as a groundline, which could denote some feelings of uncertainty and a lack of stability within her family environment (Burns & Kaufman, 1972). In addition to this, Elizabeth had drawn herself as the largest figure, which may relate to her maternal role within the family. In accordance with this, Elizabeth referred to herself as being the one to keep the family held together at various points in her life.

It may be important to note that developmentally, Elizabeth appears to be between the late Schematic Stage and the early Gang Age (around 10 years of age). At this point the writer asked Elizabeth to talk about any changes in the family dynamic when her stepsister was born because Elizabeth would have been 10 years old. Elizabeth went on to say that at this point her whole family changed. Because it was her father's first biological child and her parent's first child together, Elizabeth felt that the attention in the family shifted to focus on the new children. At the same time, she also felt the financial burden of having five children in the family and as a result, often went without. Elizabeth still seems to harbor some anger toward her mother because of how the family changed. Elizabeth placed her self and her sister, Laurelle, on one side of the table and her three half-siblings on the other side, which appeared to reinforce the separation between family members. It may be of interest to note that the table was drawn first, placing emphasis on the object as a perceived barrier between various family members. Elizabeth portrayed all members of the family with their hands and lower arms hidden under the table, which may indicate a lack of control over the environment (Burns & Kaufman, 1972).

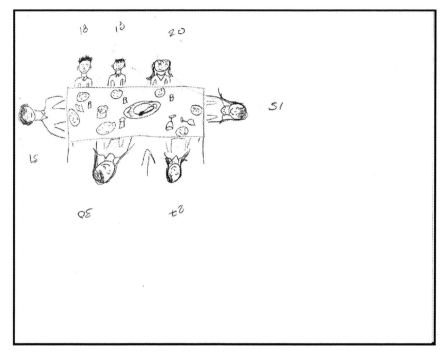

Figure 8.7. Elizabeth's KFD Response.

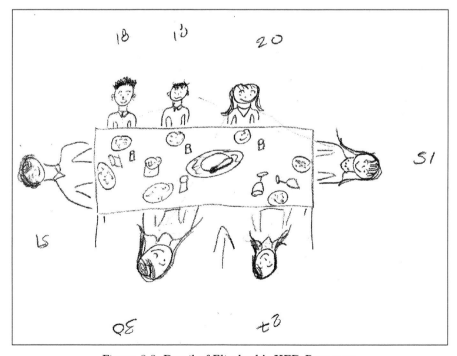

Figure 8.8. Detail of Elizabeth's KFD Response.

K-F-D ANALYSIS SHEET

Name: _Elizabeth_____   Age: _30__   Date of Birth: _6 / 9 / 78_   Sex: _Female_____

I. STYLE(S) (Circle)
- A. Compartmentalization
- B. Edging
- C. Encapsulation
- D. Folded Compartmentalization
- E. Lining on the Bottom
- F. Lining on the Top
- G. Underling individual figures

II. SYMBOL(S)

A. _____	D. _____
B. _____	E. _____
C. _____	F. _____

III. (A) ACTIONS OF INDIVIDUAL FIGURES

Figure	Action
1. Self	
2. Mother	
3. Father	
4. Older Brother	
5. Older Sister	
6. Younger Brother	
7. Younger Sister	
8. Other (Specify)	Avoidance- barrier between family

(B) ACTIONS BETWEEN INDIVIDUAL FIGURES

Figure	Action	Recipient
1. Self	Barriers	3 younger siblings
2. Mother		
3. Father		
4. O.B.		
5. O.S.		
6. Y.B.		
7. Y.S.		

IV. CHARACTERISTICS OF K-F-D FIGURES

A. Arm Extensions
1. Self	5. O.S.
2. Mother	6. Y.B.
3. Father	7. Y.S.
4. O.B.	8. Other

B. Elevated Figures
1. Self	5. O.S.
2. Mother	6. Y.B.s
3. Father	7. Y.S.
4. O.B.	8. Other

C. Erasures
1. Self	5. O.S.
2. Mother	6. Y.B.
3. Father	7. Y.S.
4. O.B.	8. Other

D. Figures on Back
1. Self	5. O.S.
2. Mother	6. Y.B.
3. Father	7. Y.S.

E. Hanging
1. Self	5. O.S.
2. Mother	6. Y.B.
3. Father	7. Y.S.
4. O.B.	8. Other

B. Location of Self

C. Distance of Self From:
Mother _2 ½ inches____   Brothers __1 inch__
Father _3/4 inch____   Sister _1 inch__

F. Omission of Body Parts
1. Self	5. O.S.
2. Mother	6. Y.B.
3. Father	7. Y.S.
4. O.B.	8. Other

G. Omission of Figures
1. Self	5. O.S.
2. Mother	6. Y.B.
3. Father	7. Y.S.
4. O.B.	8. Other

H. Picasso Eyes
1. Self	5. O.S.
2. Mother	6. Y.B.
3. Father	7. Y.S.
4. O.B.	8. Other

I. Rotated Figures
1. Self	5. O.S.
2. Mother	6. Y.B.
3. Father	7. Y.S.
4. O.B.	8. Other

V. K-F-D Grid
A. Height
1. Self _1"_ 5.Y.S. _3/4_
2. M. _1"_ 6. Y.B. _3/4_
3. F. _1 ½_ 7. Y.S. _1"_
4. O.B. ____ 8. Other ____

Figure 8.9. Elizabeth's KFD Analysis Sheet.

Example

K-F-D ANALYSIS SHEET

Name: _____ Age: _____ Date of Birth: ___ / ___ / ___ Sex: _____

I. STYLE (S) (Circle)
A. Compartmentalization
B. Edging
C. Encapsulation
D. Folded Compartmentalization
E. Lining on the Bottom
F. Lining on the Top
G. Underling individual figures

II. SYMBOL (S)
A. _____ D. _____
B. _____ E. _____
C. _____ F. _____

III. (A) ACTIONS OF INDIVIDUAL FIGURES

Figure	Action
1. Self	
2. Mother	
3. Father	
4. Older Brother	
5. Older Sister	
6. Younger Brother	
7. Younger Sister	
8. Other (Specify)	

(B) ACTIONS BETWEEN INDIVIDUAL FIGURES

Figure	Action	Recipient
1. Self		
2. Mother		
3. Father		
4. O.B.		
5. O.S.		
6. Y.B.		
7. Y.S.		
8. Other		

IV. CHARACTERISTICS OF K-F-D FIGURES

A. Arm Extensions
1. Self   5. O.S.
2. Mother   6. Y.B.
3. Father   7. Y.S.
4. O.B. 8. Other

B. Elevated Figures
1. Self   5. O.S.
2. Mother   6. Y.B.
3. Father   7. Y.S.
4. O.B. 8. Other

C. Erasures
1. Self   5. O.S.
2. Mother   6. Y.B.
3. Father   7. Y.S.
4. O.B. 8. Other

D. Figures on Back
1. Self   5. O.S.
2. Mother   6. Y.B.
3. Father   7. Y.S.
4. O.B. 8. Other

E. Hanging
1. Self   5. O.S.
2. Mother   6. Y.B.
3. Father   7. Y.S.
4. O.B. 8. Other

F. Omission of Body Parts
1. Self   5. O.S.
2. Mother   6. Y.B.
3. Father   7. Y.S.
4. O.B.   8. Other

G. Omission of Figures
1. Self   5. O.S.
2. Mother   6. Y.B.
3. Father   7. Y.S.
4. O.B.   8. Other

H. Picasso Eyes
1. Self   5. O.S.
2. Mother   6. Y.B.
3. Father   7. Y.S.
4. O.B.   8. Other

I. Rotated Figures
1. Self   5. O.S.
2. Mother   6. Y.B.
3. Father   7. Y.S.
4. O.B.   8. Other

V. K-F-D Grid

A. Height
1. Self   5. O.S.
2. M.   6. Y.B.
3. F.   7. Y.S.
4. O.B.   8. Other

B. Location of Self

C. Distance of Self From:
Mother _____ Brother _____
Father _____ Sister _____
Other (Specify) _____

KFD Grid Sheet

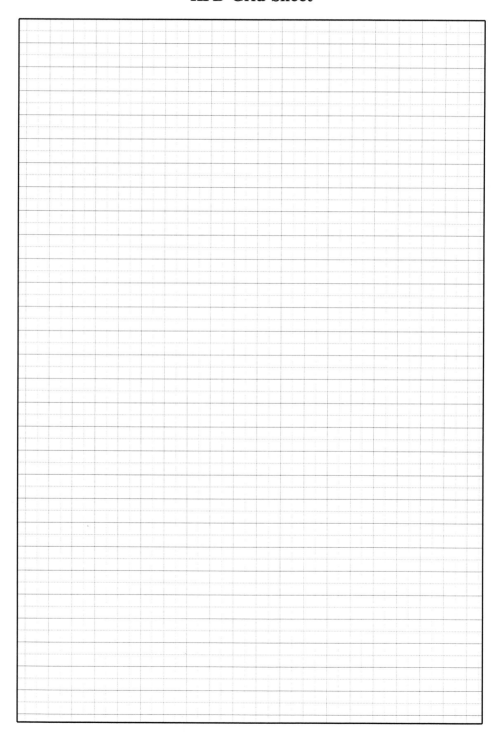

Chapter 9

PERSON PICKING AN APPLE FROM A TREE ASSESSMENT (PPAT)

Gantt and Tabone (1998) created a new instrument called the PPAT (Person Picking an Apple from A Tree) that includes the FEATS (Formal Elements Art Therapy Scale) as the rating instrument for the assessment. The manual was written to provide a method for deciphering and understanding the nonsymbolic aspects of art. The authors' intent was to formulate the structural characteristics on diagnosis and the IP's clinical state. The primary focus of the instrument was fashioned to witness *how* people drew as opposed to hone in on *what* they drew. As well, in Chapter 6 of Gantt and Tabone's manual the focal point was placed on "pattern matching;" that is to distinguish the differences between the four classic Axis I disorders (major depression, schizophrenia, organic mental disorders, and bipolar disorder) as correlated with the FEATS (Gantt & Tabone, 1998, p. 26) scales. For example:

Axis I	DSM Symptom	Art Therapy Literature	Feats Scale
Major Depression	Loss of energy; psychomotor retardation or agitation	Constricted use of space	#3 Energy #4 Space

In this venue, Gantt and Tabone have attempted to correlate the responses (or lack thereof) to the observable behavior and PPAT artwork of the IP. As well, the content scales (in Chapter 5) and tally sheets provided in the Appendix section of their book highlights information about explicit color use, anomalies (adding writing or numbers), and specific ecological and clothing particulars.

When using the FEATS in its entirety (which these authors recommend), one should include the following information when the imparted rating and content tally sheets are used for a thesis, dissertation and/or publication:

> The Formal Elements Art Scale, copyright© 1990, 1998 by Linda Gantt, is used [or reproduced] by written permission of Gargoyle Press, 314 Scott Avenue, Morgantown, WV 26508.

Moreover, it is recommended that this copyright information be included in formal art therapy assessment evaluations and that all content and tally sheets be adhered to the Appendix of an Art Therapy Assessment, should the reader of the evaluative material want more information. As Gantt and Tabone (1998) point out, the "ultimate aim of diagnosis should be to inform treatment decisions" (p. 3).

The idea of cogently summarizing information and transliterating that back to other mental health clinicians, health care and/or medical practitioners is the utmost aim of this book and therefore Gantt and Tabone's adage exactly mirrors the scope of this book.

Historically, a person picking an apple from a tree (or the PPAT) was first described by Viktor Lowenfeld (1939, 1947). This was featured in a study he conducted on children's use of space in art. His instructions were more detailed than Gantt and Tabone's method (1998) and were as follows:

> You are under a tree. On one of its branches you see an apple that you particularly admire and that you would like to have. You stretch out your hand to pick the apple, but your reach is a little short. Then you make a great effort and get the apple after all. Now you have it and enjoy eating it. Draw yourself as you are taking the apple off the tree. (1947, pp. 75–76)

Gantt and Tabone (1998) suggested that the subject be offered 12 x 18 inch white drawing paper and 12 colors of felt-tip markers (red, orange, blue, turquoise, green, dark green, hot pink, magenta, purple, brown, yellow, and black) offered as the scented Sanford® "Mr. Sketch."® (The participant, not the administrant, decides the orientation of the drawing paper.) Early on, the test was conducted using pastels but a number of participants expressed dissatisfaction with the medium. While markers limit expressiveness, the materials were used because of ease to count colors used and ease of information provided. Directions are simply to hand the paper to the subject and simply say, "Draw a person picking an apple from a tree." If asked about gender, the above sentence is repeated with the emphasis on the word "person." There is no time limit on completion of the task. Should apples not grow on trees (if subjects are from countries where apples do not grow on trees), it is suggested that any tree/fruit combination be used in lieu of the word "apple." Cross-cultural studies were of less interest to Gantt and Tabone (1998) than the problem-solving abilities of the participant (p. 16).

The actual FEATS scale offers a range of possible responses with five points on each scale (rather than simply the presence or absence of a characteristic). As well the administrant can mark anywhere along the continuum line of zero (for example no representation of color) to five (indicating color used to outline forms, objects, and fill in space – e.g., completely colored sky). The rater can also mark in between noting subtleties such as 2.5. There are a total of 14 art therapy scale items that are rated (see Appendix of Gantt & Tabone, 1998). The FEATS scale has a total best possible score of 70 points.

There is also a tally content sheet covering the orientation of the picture, colors used in the whole picture/person, color used for person/gender, actual energy of the person, orientation of person's face, approximate age of person/clothing/apple tree, color of apple tree, environmental details, and other features (see Appendix of Gantt & Tabone, 1998). The tally sheet is merely a check sheet.

Below are examples of the PPAT on clients with varying etiologies. The authors redirect the reader to the Gantt and Tabone (1998) source for additional information, research and sample discussions.

Identified Patient: Holly

DOB: 1978

CA: 27

Testing Dates: April 2, 2006

Administrant: Jane C. Adams
Assessments Administered: ATDA, HTP, PPAT

See Chapters 2 and 7 for further examples regarding Holly.

Refer to Appendix A for Genogram, Timeline, Behavioral Observations, and Psychosocial Indicators.

The purpose of the Formal Element Art Therapy Scale (FEATS) seems to be to identify characteristics of a client's drawing, which fall outside a perceived normal or standard way of producing the directed picture. Structural characteristics provide information about the client's current psychological state, which may not be visible through other means. The FEATS is applied to the drawing known as the Person Picking an Apple from a Tree (PPAT).

The purpose of the scale is research and information collection. Gantt and Tabone (1998) developed this scoring method based on the DSM-IV-TR, on their clinical observations, and on assessment literature available at the time. According to Betts (2005), the number of assessment instruments is so large and the supporting literature so voluminous as to confuse the identification of the best or most appropriate tools for specific application. The FEATS has adequate statistical data backing it up that it appears to be among the most useful of the art therapy assessments. This writer has collected data from Holly and completed both the FEATS and Content Tally Sheets.

In the FEATS, Holly scored at the high end of the scale in most of the 14 characteristics. This would be consistent with her attainment of Horovitz's (2002) Artistic Stage. Holly's PPAT drawing included a prominence of color, good color fit, and demonstrates her ability to problem-solve and apply logic. Her drawing is well-integrated with good line quality and use of space. She shows no perseveration or rotation and seems to be in full control of her drawing.

Repeating the assessment again may allow identification of some change as in the HTP subtests (see Chapter 7) which reflected some potentially significant differences between the first (chromatic) and second (achromatic) assessments. High total score on the FEATS may indicate that Holly is not a fit with the typical population groups most often used as control groups with the FEATS.

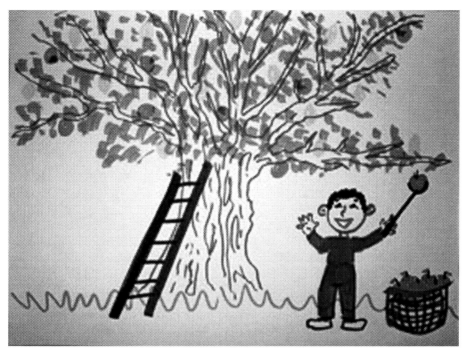

Figure 9.1. Holly's PPAT Response. (For color version, see Plate 24, p. 120.)

Conclusion

Holly possibly has issues and inner personal conflict, which may be creating anxiety and frustration for her. All of her assessment results appear to indicate a set of unresolved issues. These seem to be related to her need for privacy and her struggle to cope with intimacy. Her drawings seem to indicate that she has achieved a measure of maturity visible in reaching Horovitz's (2002) Artistic Stage. Yet she remains stuck in Freud's Anal Stage of psychosexual development. She appears to be conflicted in her relationship with her family, both needing their attention and retreating from their presence.

Recommendations

To deal with her intimacy issues, the writer suggests a series of group art therapy sessions in order to develop the skills Holly might need to cope with and to succeed in family art therapy. The writer also recommends that Holly pursue a course of family art therapy.

Identified Patient: S

DOB: 2000

CA: 6 years old

Testing Dates: February 26, 2006; March 6, 2006; March 27, 2006

Administrant: Jacob Atkinson

Assessments Administered: CATA, PPAT, SDT

See Chapters 1, 5, and 10 for further examples regarding S.

Refer to Appendix A for Genogram, Timeline, Behavioral Observations, and Psychosocial Indicators.

S was handed a white 12" x 18" sheet of paper, along with the appropriate markers assigned to the PPAT. S was then instructed to "Draw a person picking an apple from a tree." The administrant utilized the FEATS rating and content tally sheets (see Figures 9.3–9.6). S's overall rating score was a 52.5 out of a possible 70, and she falls into the FEATS nonpatient Grouping (Gantt & Tabone, 1998). In her drawing S has made the apple overly large and orange. This overemphasis on the size of the fruit may again be a sign of her need for increased nurturance both physically and emotionally. Though the girl in the drawing has to lean and reach quite far for the apple, her ladder appears stable enough to support her imbalanced position. Only half of the nurture-giving tree is shown, which may imply poor planning. This may also suggest that she is only receiving the nurturance she needs from one parent, as there is only half a tree and one apple to choose from. Also, there are no roots connecting the tree to the groundline, which may indicate repressed emotions (Oster & Crone, 2004).

Conclusion and Recommendations

S is a bright child whose overall artistic response is within Lowenfeld & Brittain's Schematic Stage. She displays attributes in her art that suggest a need for nurturance, warmth, and love, as displayed by her overly large apple and TV. Hammer (1980) also suggests that individuals who have digestive disturbances may draw figures with elongated necks, which is congruent with S's art and physical diagnosis. This administrator recommends continued art therapy for S as she seems to enjoy art but more importantly can communicate her feelings through art. Continued sessions will allow S the opportunity to learn appropriate strategies for coping with and expressing her feelings. Also sessions involving the family in the future are recommended to help bring S's need for increased emotional nurturance to the attention of her family.

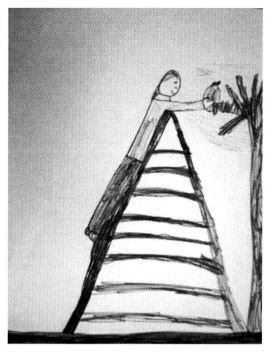

Figure 9.2. S's PPAT Response. (For color version, see Plate 25, p. 121.)

Picture #: _1_

Rater: _JAKE_

FORMAL ELEMENTS ART THERAPY SCALE (FEATS)©
RATING SHEET

Linda Gantt, Ph.D., ATR-BC, & Carmello Tabone, M.A., ATR

The FEATS uses scales that measure **more or less** of the particular variable. Look at the degree to which a picture fits the particular scale by comparing the picture you are rating with the examples in the illustrated rating manual. **You may mark between the numbers on the scales.** Approach the picture as if you did not know what it was supposed to be. Can you recognize individual items? If you have a picture that is hard to rate, do your best to compare it to the illustrations and the written descriptions. Do not worry whether your rating is the same as another rater's. Concentrate on giving your first impression to the variable being measured.

#1 - Prominence of Color

| Color used for outlining only | 0   1   2   3   ④   5 | Color used to fill all available space |

#2 - Color Fit

| Colors not related to task | 0   1   2   3   ④   5 | Colors related to task |

#3 - Implied energy

| No energy | 0   1   2   ③   4   5 | Excessive energy |

#4 - Space

| Less than 25% of space used | 0   1   2   3 ③ 4   5 | 100% of space used |

#5 - Integration

| Not at all integrated | 0   1   2   3 ④ 5 | Fully integrated |

#6 - Logic

| Entire picture is bizarre or illogical | 0   1   2   3   4   ⑤ | Picture is logical |

From: L. Gantt & C. Tabone, 1998, *The Formal Elements Art Therapy Scale: The Rating Manual*, Morgantown, WV: Gargoyle Press. Copyright © 1998 Linda Gantt.

Figure 9.3a. S's FEATS Rating Sheet I.

#7 - Realism

Not realistic (cannot
tell what was drawn)
0 | 1 | 2 | ③ | 4 | 5
Quite realistic

#8 - Problem-solving

No evidence of
problem-solving
0 | 1 | 2 | 3 | 4 | ⑤
Reasonable solution
to picking apple

#9 - Developmental Level

Two-year-old
level
0 | 1 | 2 | ③ | 4 | 5
Adult level

#10 - Details of Objects and Environment

No details or
environment
0 | 1 | 2 ② 3 | 4 | 5
Full environment,
abundant details

#11 - Line Quality

Broken, "damaged"
lines
0 | 1 | 2 | ③ | 4 | 5
Fluid, flowing
lines

#12 - Person

No person
depicted
0 | 1 | 2 | 3 | 4 ④ 5
Realistic person

#13 - Rotation

Pronounced
rotation
0 | 1 | 2 | 3 | ④ | 5
Trees & people,
upright, no rotation

#14 - Perseveration

Severe
0 | 1 | 2 | 3 | ④ | 5
None

From: L. Gantt & C. Tabone, 1998, *The Formal Elements Art Therapy Scale: The Rating Manual*,
Morgantown, WV: Gargoyle Press. Copyright © 1998 Linda Gantt.

Figure 9.3b. S's FEATS Rating Sheet II.

CONTENT TALLY SHEET
"Draw a Person Picking an Apple from a Tree"

Picture #: <u>1</u>
Rater: <u>JAKE</u>

Instructions for Coding: Approach the picture as if you did not know what it was supposed to be. Can you recognize the individual items? Place a check for all items you see in the picture. If there is no category for an item try to describe it in the section called "Other Features" (Section 13). If there are two or more persons in the picture designate the person on the left as Person #1, the next person to the right as Person #2, and so on.

1. Orientation of Picture

Horizontal		Vertical	✗

2. Colors Used in the Whole Picture
(Check all colors used)

Blue	✓	Turquoise	
Red	✓	Purple	
Green	✓	Dark green	✓
Brown	✓	Black	
Pink	✓	Magenta	✓
Orange	✓	Yellow	

3. Person (If this is marked skip to Section #9.)

Cannot identify any part of the drawing as a person	
(If this is marked, score Section #3 & 8)	
Only arm or hand seen reaching for or grasping apple	

4. Color Used for Person
Check all colors used for the person(s) (or arm or hand) including the clothes. If you cannot identify the person do not code this section.

	Person #1	#2	#3
Blue	✓		
Turquoise			
Red	✓		
Green			
Dark green			
Brown	✓		
Black			
Purple			
Pink	✓		
Magenta	✓		
Orange			
Yellow			

5. Gender

	Person #1	#2	#3
Cannot tell (ambiguous or stick figure)			
Definitely male			
Might be male			
Definitely female	✓		
Might be female			

6. Actual Energy of Person
(The categories are not mutually exclusive - ex., person could be sitting <u>and</u> reaching toward apple.)

	Person #1	#2	#3
Prone			
Sitting			
Standing on implied or actual ground			
Standing on box, ladder, or other object	✓		
Reaching toward nothing			
Reaching down or up toward apple or object			
Floating (feet higher than base of tree with no groundline or visible support for feet)			
Hanging (appears suspended from tree or branch)			
Jumping up (may have "action lines")			
Jumping or falling out of tree			
Climbing tree without ladder			
Flying			
Other (if you cannot use one of the above categories describe it as best you can):			

7. Orientation of Person's Face
How much can you see of the person's face?

	Person #1	#2	#3
Cannot tell			
Front view - no features			
Front view with at least one feature (ex., eyes)			
Profile	✓		
Three-quarters view			
Back of head			

8. Approximate Age of Person

	Person #1	#2	#3
Cannot tell (ambiguous or stick figure)			
Baby or child			
Adolescent or adult	✓		

Figure 9.4a. S's Content Tally Sheet I.

9. Clothing

	Person	#1	#2	#3
Hat				
No clothes (stick figure or hand)				
Nude				
Some suggestion of clothes (may be a line indicating neckline or hem; may be same color as person; may be a sleeve or suggestion of sleeve if only hand is shown)				
Well-drawn clothes done in different colors than person (ex., street clothes or work clothes, dress, jumpsuit)		/		
Costume (specify):				

10. Apple Tree

If you cannot identify any part as an apple tree, a branch, or a stem, check the first box and skip to Section #11. Count the total number of apples you can see, whether they are in the person's hand, on the ground, in the tree, or in a container.

No identifiable apple tree or branch or stem	
Only one apple in the picture:	▉
Only a stem or branch with one apple on it, no tree trunk	
Trunk and top visible (may run off edge of paper) with one apple	/
2-10 apples	
More than 10 apples	
Apples placed on perimeter of top*	

* Code if the apples are placed around edge of tree top, on stems sticking out from edge of top, or only at the ends of branches rather than in the tree.

11. Color of Apple Tree

Trunk:	
Brown	/
Black	
Other (specify):	
Top (may be distinct leaves or lollipop top or rounded form):	▉
Green and/or dark green	/
Other (specify):	
Apples:	▉
Red	
Yellow	
Green/dark green	
Other (specify): *orange*	/

12. Environmental Details

If you cannot identify any details in the categories below check the first box and skip to Section #12.

No identifiable environmental details	
Natural details:	▉
Sun, sunrise, sunset	
Moon	
Grass or horizon line	/
Flowers	
Tree (other than apple tree)	
Clouds, rain, wind	
Mountains or hills	
Lake or pond	
Stream, river, or creek	
Sky (filled in or sky line)	
Rainbow	
Animals:	▉
Dog	
Cat	
Bird	
Cow, sheep, farm animal	
Butterflies	
Other (specify):	
Imaginary items, machines, or animals (specify):	
Inanimate items:	▉
Fence	
Sign	
House	
Walkway, path or road	
Car, truck, or wagon	
Other (specify):	
Ladders	/
Baskets, boxes, or containers	
Apple pickers or sticks	
Other (specify):	

13. Other Features

Writing (not a signature or on a sign)	
Numbers (not a date or on a sign)	
Geometric shape(s)	
Seemingly random marks	
Other (specify):	

Figure 9.4b. S's Content Tally Sheet II.

Identified Patient: L

DOB: January 20, 1958

CA: 49

Testing Date: April 1, 2007

Administrant: Barbara Murak

Assessments Administered: ATDA, BATA, PPAT

See Chapters 2 and 3 for further examples regarding L.

Refer to Appendix A for Genogram, Timeline, Behavioral Observations, and Psychosocial Indicators.

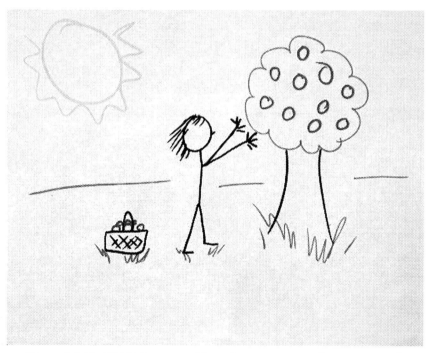

Figure 9.5. L's PPAT Response. (For color version, see Plate 26, p. 121.)

The client chose a horizontal orientation for her drawing and drew in black a child-like, rigid stick figure. The rigid stance and averted head suggest an inflexibility of reaction, a tendency to avoid facing issues squarely, and rigidity in her relationship with people in general (Hammer, 1980). Additional materials drawn were a sun and a basket containing apples. The sun was added last, with client stating "that should warm up things" possibly indicating client's feelings of longing for warmth from her environment (Hammer, 1980). The client's stick figure, child-like drawing could be attributed to her initial tension and anxiety (Hammer, 1980).

Point Value for colors were:

1. Prominence of Color: 1 – color is only used to outline forms and objects.
2. Color Fit: 3 – some color, but not all, are used appropriately.
3. Implied Energy: 2.5 – relatively little energy – average amount.
4. Space: 4 – approximately 75% of the space is used.
5. Integration: 2 – a visual relationship between 2 elements.
6. Logic: 5 – no bizarre or illogical elements in the picture.
7. Realism: 2 – items are recognizable but simply drawn.
8. Problem-Solving: 4 – person is on the ground and is reaching for apple.
9. Developmental Level: 2.5 – like those of 4–6 year-old; arms appear to be coming from neck.
10. Details of Objects & Environment: 3 – horizon line and 1–2 details.
11. Line Quality: 4 – lines are under control.
12. Person: 3 – the person is drawn as a stick figure with at least a circle for the head.
13. Rotation: 5 – there is no rotation; person and tree are vertical.
14. Perseveration: 5 – there is no perseveration.

Assessment Results

Based on the Pre-Test Mood Questionnaire, the client presented as relaxed and in a good mood (5), not uncomfortable (1), feeling positive (5), and not stressed and overwhelmed (1). These scores did not differ upon completion of the FEATS assessment. In addition, the client and this writer wore squares of "stress tabs" visibly on our foreheads. Both remained blue for the entire 2-hour assessment session. Although the client's mood answers did not differ, her blood pressure readings did. Her Systolic reading dropped 6 points, and the Diastolic dropped 10 points (104/65, pulse 66 – 98/55, pulse 60). The client mentioned her readings are "normally very low." Just prior to the blood pressure reading, the client stood up and pulled her sweater off over her head and said, "I love taking off my clothes. Oh wait! This is not a date, this is an art assessment." This initiates a theme of the client's sexual preoccupation. The client completed her assessments after a weekend of dating and sex. The timing of collection is crucial (Gantt & Tabone, 1998).

The client's scores on the FEATS suggest depression, as seen in the nude, black-drawn stick figure, general lack of environmental details, and color used only for outlining (Gantt & Tabone, 1998). The client provided few details, but appropriate. Gantt & Tabone (1998) state that the drawings of people with major depression show the problem-solving process as adequate, with the person usually shown reaching for the apple, yet not grasping one. In depressed responses, the person is often drawn as a stick figure (Gantt & Tabone, 1998). It should also be noted that the client disclosed she ceased treatment for depression one year ago, and currently is not in psychotherapy, nor on any antidepressant medication. Her last treatment was three years in length and Zoloft was prescribed.

Conclusions

The client's childlike drawings could indicate that in periods of stress, she regresses to the developmental age range preceding that period in her life when she was starved for emotional nourishment from her environment, perhaps preadolescent (Hammer, 1980). Her numerous dating and sexual encounters would indicate that the client is longing to experience nurturing, emotional warmth, and interpersonal relationships that were lacking in her childhood. The client seems to be experiencing conflicted feelings of rigidity and lack of control regarding her sexual impulses. This writer would recommend further art therapy to address issues of loneliness, depression, self-esteem, insecurity, and fear of contamination as a result of her promiscuity. All drawings began at the right-hand side of the paper, which may indicate inhibition. Rigidity of her self-drawings indicate keeping herself closed off against the world, while simultaneously keeping her inner impulses under rigid control (Hammer, 1980).

Picture #: *1*

Rater: *B. MURAK*

FORMAL ELEMENTS ART THERAPY SCALE (FEATS)©
RATING SHEET

Linda Gantt, Ph.D., ATR-BC, & Carmello Tabone, M.A., ATR

The FEATS uses scales that measure **more or less** of the particular variable. Look at the degree to which a picture fits the particular scale by comparing the picture you are rating with the examples in the illustrated rating manual. **You may mark between the numbers on the scales.** Approach the picture as if you did not know what it was supposed to be. Can you recognize individual items? If you have a picture that is hard to rate, do your best to compare it to the illustrations and the written descriptions. Do not worry whether your rating is the same as another rater's. Concentrate on giving your first impression to the variable being measured.

#1 - Prominence of Color

Color used for outlining only   0 | (1) | 2 | 3 | 4 | 5   Color used to fill all available space

---

#2 - Color Fit

Colors not related to task   0 | 1 | 2 | (3) | 4 | 5   Colors related to task

---

#3 - Implied energy

No energy   0 | 1 | 2 (|) 3 | 4 | 5   Excessive energy

#4 - Space

Less than 25% of space used   0 | 1 | 2 | 3 | (4) | 5   100% of space used

---

#5 - Integration

Not at all integrated   0 | 1 | (2) | 3 | 4 | 5   Fully integrated

---

#6 - Logic

Entire picture is bizarre or illogical   0 | 1 | 2 | 3 | 4 | (5)   Picture is logical

---

Figure 9.6a. L's FEATS Rating Sheet I.

#7 - Realism

Not realistic (cannot   0 | 1 | (2) | 3 | 4 | 5   Quite realistic
tell what was drawn)

#8 - Problem-solving

No evidence of   0 | 1 | 2 | 3 | (4) | 5   Reasonable solution
problem-solving   to picking apple

#9 - Developmental Level

Two-year-old   0 | 1 | 2 (1) 3 | 4 | 5   Adult level
level

#10 - Details of Objects and Environment

No details or   0 | 1 | 2 | (3) | 4 | 5   Full environment,
environment   abundant details

#11 - Line Quality

Broken, "damaged"   0 | 1 | 2 | 3 | (4) | 5   Fluid, flowing
lines   lines

#12 - Person

No person   0 | 1 | 2 | (3) | 4 | 5   Realistic person
depicted

#13 - Rotation

Pronounced   0 | 1 | 2 | 3 | 4 | (5)   Trees & people,
rotation   upright, no rotation

#14 - Perseveration

Severe   0 | 1 | 2 | 3 | 4 | (5)   None

From: L. Gantt & C. Tabone, 1998, *The Formal Elements Art Therapy Scale: The Rating Manual,*
Morgantown, WV: Gargoyle Press. Copyright © 1998 Linda Gantt.

Figure 9.6b. L's FEATS Rating Sheet II.

CONTENT TALLY SHEET
"Draw a Person Picking an Apple from a Tree"

Picture #: 1
Rater: P. MURAK

Instructions for Coding: Approach the picture as if you did not know what it was supposed to be. Can you recognize the individual items? Place a check for all items you see in the picture. If there is no category for an item try to describe it in the section called "Other Features" (Section 13). If there are two or more persons in the picture designate the person on the left as Person #1, the next person to the right as Person #2, and so on.

1. Orientation of Picture

Horizontal	X	Vertical	

2. Colors Used in the Whole Picture
(Check all colors used)

Blue	X	Turquoise	
Red	X	Purple	
Green	X	Dark green	
Brown	X	Black	
Pink		Magenta	
Orange		Yellow	X

3. Person (If this is marked skip to Section #9.)

Cannot identify any part of the drawing as a person	
(If this is marked, score Section #3 & 8)	
Only arm or hand seen reaching for or grasping apple	

4. Color Used for Person
Check all colors used for the person(s) (or arm or hand) including the clothes. If you cannot identify the person do not code this section.

Person	#1	#2	#3
Blue			
Turquoise			
Red			
Green			
Dark green			
Brown			
Black	X		
Purple			
Pink			
Magenta			
Orange			
Yellow			

5. Gender

Person	#1	#2	#3
Cannot tell (ambiguous or stick figure)			
Definitely male			
Might be male			
Definitely female			
Might be female	X		

6. Actual Energy of Person
(The categories are not mutually exclusive - ex., person could be sitting and reaching toward apple.)

Person	#1	#2	#3
Prone			
Sitting			
Standing on implied or actual ground	X		
Standing on box, ladder, or other object			
Reaching toward nothing			
Reaching down or up toward apple or object	X		
Floating (feet higher than base of tree with no groundline or visible support for feet)			
Hanging (appears suspended from tree or branch)			
Jumping up (may have "action lines")			
Jumping or falling out of tree			
Climbing tree without ladder			
Flying			
Other (if you cannot use one of the above categories describe it as best you can):			

7. Orientation of Person's Face
How much can you see of the person's face?

Person	#1	#2	#3
Cannot tell			
Front view - no features			
Front view with at least one feature (ex., eyes)			
Profile	X		
Three-quarters view			
Back of head			

8. Approximate Age of Person

Person	#1	#2	#3
Cannot tell (ambiguous or stick figure)	X		
Baby or child			
Adolescent or adult			

Figure 9.7a. L's Content Tally Sheet I.

9. Clothing

	Person	#1	#2	#3
Hat				
No clothes (stick figure or hand)		X		
Nude				
Some suggestion of clothes (may be a line indicating neckline or hem; may be same color as person; may be a sleeve or suggestion of sleeve if only hand is shown)				
Well-drawn clothes done in different colors than person (ex., street clothes or work clothes, dress, jumpsuit)				
Costume (specify):				

10. Apple Tree

If you cannot identify any part as an apple tree, a branch, or a stem, check the first box and skip to Section #11. Count the total number of apples you can see, whether they are in the person's hand, on the ground, in the tree, or in a container.

No identifiable apple tree or branch or stem	
Only one apple in the picture:	■
Only a stem or branch with one apple on it, no tree trunk	
Trunk and top visible (may run off edge of paper) with one apple	
2-10 apples	
More than 10 apples	X
Apples placed on perimeter of top*	

* Code if the apples are placed around edge of tree top, on stems sticking out from edge of top, or only at the ends of branches rather than in the tree.

11. Color of Apple Tree

Trunk:	■
Brown	X
Black	
Other (specify):	
Top (may be distinct leaves or lollipop top or rounded form):	■
Green and/or dark green	X
Other (specify):	
Apples:	■
Red	X
Yellow	
Green/dark green	
Other (specify):	

12. Environmental Details

If you cannot identify any details in the categories below check the first box and skip to Section #12.

No identifiable environmental details	
Natural details:	■
Sun, sunrise, sunset	X
Moon	
Grass or horizon line	X
Flowers	
Tree (other than apple tree)	
Clouds, rain, wind	
Mountains or hills	
Lake or pond	
Stream, river, or creek	
Sky (filled in or sky line)	
Rainbow	
Animals:	■
Dog	
Cat	
Bird	
Cow, sheep, farm animal	
Butterflies	
Other (specify):	
Imaginary items, machines, or animals (specify):	
Inanimate items:	■
Fence	
Sign	
House	
Walkway, path or road	
Car, truck, or wagon	
Other (specify):	
Ladders	
Baskets, boxes, or containers	X
Apple pickers or sticks	
Other (specify):	

13. Other Features

Writing (not a signature or on a sign)	
Numbers (not a date or on a sign)	
Geometric shape(s)	
Seemingly random marks	
Other (specify):	

Figure 9.7b. L's Content Tally Sheet II.

Identified Patient: Sandy

DOB: May 23, 1972

CA: 33

Testing Date: April 9, 2006

Administrant: Rachel N. Sikorski

Assessments Administered: CATA, FSA, PPAT

See Chapters 5 and 6 for further examples regarding Sandy.

Refer to Appendix A for Genogram, Timeline, Behavioral Observations, and Psychosocial Indicators.

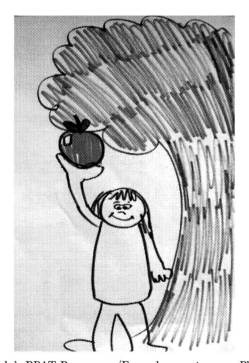

Figure 9.8. Sandy's PPAT Response. (For color version, see Plate 27, p. 122.)

Sandy began this task by using a black marker to create the outline of a tree, which appears to go off the right side as well as crowds the top of the drawing page. She filled in the trunk and crown of the tree with large, quick strokes of color, using brown and green, respectively. Sandy chose black once again to create the outline of an apple, a hand, and a standing figure. She finished by coloring in the apple with red and the apple leaves and stem with green.

Sandy drew large shapes on a piece of paper that was vertically oriented, and in doing so, the tree appeared to extend beyond the border of the drawing page. This could be an indicator of poor planning, and it is likely a sign of Sandy's anxiety and a lack of confidence in her artistic abilities. Moreover, because the tree seems to cling to the edge of the paper and there is no indication of a root structure on Sandy's tree, it may reflect a potential need for stability or support. The apparent lack of a branch system in her tree may point to a potential need for control when making contacts with the environment (Hammer, 1980). Although Sandy used naturalistic color choices for the tree, the colors may further indicate the need for control (green) or repression of emotions (brown) (Hammer, 1980). The line quality of the three main, colored-in forms (trunk, crown, and apple) suggest hurriedness or perhaps some anxiety with completing the task.

Sandy's figure was left uncolored, but is facing the viewer with apparent confidence and seems to have successfully picked an apple. The visibility of the tree through the figure's feet could be a sign of Sandy's immaturity, and according to the FEATS scale, she seems to be functioning at the latency age developmental level (Gantt & Tabone, 1998). The diametrically opposed feet of Sandy's drawn figure might indicate instability or ambiguity; however, despite this fact, the feet appear to be solid on the ground and therefore suggest stability (Oster & Crone, 2004). Hammer (1980) states that the drawing of a sturdy tree often shows a strong similarity to the person drawn, and in this case, they both seem to be standing solid and determined.

Sandy scored a 50.5 out of a possible 70 points on the FEATS rating scale, which points to the likelihood that she is functioning as a nonpatient. Although Sandy used little color and detail, a high level of energy could be seen in the line quality and expansive use of space, and she showed her ability to problem-solve successfully (Gantt & Tabone, 1998).

Recommendations and Conclusion

Sandy's responses to the Face Stimulus Drawing, PPAT, and CATA assessments may reflect anxiety, a lack of confidence, and a distorted self-perception. Her family history and experience as the middle child of her family may have had an impact on her self-concept and confidence.

Sandy's expressions are simple, reserved, and quickly executed. Her role as middle child in the family, as well as her experiences of receiving less attention than her siblings, may have influenced her self-perception. The building of creativity and the promotion of self-expression that art therapy offers may be beneficial for Sandy in developing increased self-knowledge and more confidence in her abilities.

The writer recommends that Sandy consider engaging in art therapy on a regular basis, so that she may find a constructive outlet for emotional expression and develop increased self-confidence and a stronger self-concept.

FEATS results:

1. *Prominence of Color:* 3 − Black outlines, only tree and apple were colored in
2. *Color Fit:* 4 − Most colors used appropriately, person left uncolored
3. *Implied Energy:* 3 − Average energy level
4. *Space:* 4 − About 75% of space used
5. *Integration:* 4 − Visual relationship between 3 elements (tree, apple, person)
6. *Logic:* 4.5 − Generally logical, person uncolored appears slightly bizarre
7. *Realism:* 2.5 − Items recognizable, simply drawn
8. *Problem-Solving:* 5 − Person successful, grasping an apple
9. *Developmental Level:* 3 − Latency-age response, objects along a baseline
10. *Details of Objects & Environment:* 1.5 − Little detail; only person, tree, apple
11. *Line Quality:* 3 − Some continuous lines
12. *Person:* 4 − Most elements drawn, missing neck
13. *Rotation:* 5 − No rotation
14. *Perseveration:* 4 − Very little, in trunk and crown of tree

Chapter 10

SILVER DRAWING TEST (SDT)

Doctor Rawley Silver converged two vocations, that as a social worker and a painter in the 1960s. Her decision to become a social worker evolved after volunteering to teach in a school where she met "Charlie," an extraordinarily talented, hearing-impaired young man. Her work with this youngster catapulted her towards completing her degrees in fine arts and fine arts education at Columbia University (since the field of Art Therapy had not yet been officially birthed). She worked with numerous children and other adults who had varying disabilities. Her desire to understand the emotional and cognitive needs of these aforementioned populations was the seed for the Silver Drawing Test (SDT) and many other assessments outlined in her opus work, *Three Art Assessments* (Silver, 2002). Indeed, Silver's earlier works on these assessments were amongst the first batteries that were empirically tested, thus offering art therapists standing in the scientific community (Horovitz, 1985).

The SDT was designed to assess three concepts fundamental to mathematics and reading. Her work is based on the work of Jean Piaget (1967, 1970), who remains famous for his work in conservation and spatial concepts. The first subtest (Predictive Drawing) was based on the concept of a group and applied classes and numbers. It allowed for subject prediction of sequencing, horizontality and verticality. The second subtest (Drawing from Observation) was based on sequential order and applied to relationships. This subtest allowed the subject to create observable data and draft the relationships from horizontal (left-right), vertical (above-below), and depth (front-back). The final subtest (Drawing from Imagination) applied stimulus drawing ideas of space, neighborhoods, points of view, and frames of reference.

The cognitive content of the Drawing from Imagination subtest was related to the ability to select (that is the content or message behind the drawing), the ability to combine (that is the form of the drawing itself), and finally the ability to represent (the concepts and creativity of the form, content, title or story evolving from the resulting drawing). As well there are two different choices to stimulate the Drawing from Imagination responses, forms A or B, chosen at the discretion of the administrant.

Moreover, it should be noted that unlike the previous subtests, the final subtest (Drawing from Imagination) inherently produces a projective on the part of the maker. As a result three areas can be scored: (1) emotional content for strongly negative to strongly positive themes; (2) self–image for morbid fantasy to wish-fulfilling fantasy; and (3) use of humor from strongly aggressive humor to playful humor. (It should be noted that the emotive scores are not factored into the cognitive results, thus providing additional information for the clinician that he or she can use when beginning art therapy treatment.)

Note the entire *cognitive* scoring system has a 6-point system ranging from 0–5 with 5 being the best possible score for each subsection (3) of each subtest (3). Thus the best possible score is 5 on each subsection and 5 on each subtest yielding a total best score of 45.

The *emotive* scales (linked only to the Drawing from Imagination subtest and which can be used at the discretion of the administrant) are scored from 1–5 points, 5 reflecting the most positive emotive content. Again the emotive scores are *not* factored into the percentile rank and final t-score conversion is found in the normative data scales (Silver, 2002, pp. 92–96).

Finally, Horovitz's personal favorite aspect of this battery is that it can be used as a pretest/posttest for amassing cognitive gain and recovery in the client (Horovitz, 1985). As well, it is short, easy to administer, and can be readily used when working with clients who have short attention spans. Review of the entire assessment in Silver's text (2002) is highly recommended in order to completely understand the instructions and use of this test with individuals and groups.

According to Horovitz (2008), if one wanted to go *one step further* with this assessment, she encourages Silver (or future practitioners) to reproduce the results of the Drawing from Observation subtest in 3-dimensional media (preferably clay) in order to yield data that could reveal vastly different results from working with 2-dimensional media.

Following are samples of this assessment.

Identified Patient: S

DOB: 2000

CA: 6 years old

Testing Dates: February 26, 2006; March 6, 2006; March 27, 2006

Administrant: Jacob Atkinson

Assessments Administered: CATA, PPAT, SDT

See Chapters 1, 5, and 9 for further examples regarding S.

Refer to Appendix A for Genogram, Timeline, Behavioral Observations, and Psychosocial Indicators.

Predictive Drawing:	9
Drawing from Observation	8
Drawing from Imagination	12
Total Score	29

S received a total score of 29 out of 45 possible points. This overall score placed her in the 99+ percentile, with a T score of 76.39 for six to seven-year-old first graders (Silver, 2002). S was able to accurately depict sequencing in task one of the Predictive Drawing subtest. Her response to task two, of this subtest demonstrates that she has not yet acquired the ability to predict horizontality. S does have water spilling out of the jug, which in reality would occur if the second jug were as full as her first jug when tipped. Her response to the third task in the Predictive Drawing subtest shows that Susan is beginning to grasp the concept of verticality, but does not fully comprehend it. She scored in the 97 percentile for her age group in this subtest (Silver, 2002). S's second subtest, Drawing from Observation, displays that her ability to form spatial relationships is still developing. She scored in the 75 percentile for her age group in this subtest (Silver, 2002).

S's Drawing from Imagination subtest was of a cat on its back playing with a ball of string, while a dog observed the cat. In this subtest she demonstrates the ability to select, combine, and represent in the 97th percentile for her age group (Silver, 2002). It is the story that she created to accompany this image that is so telling. Her story involved the cat and dog switching attributes, and then going to the Vet. The Vet told them it was just "a case called opposite case" and that "it wasn't serious." The story has implication of her many experiences of going to doctors, and a cry for normalcy. Also implied, is the roll reversal that she may be feeling towards her mother as S has often expressed feelings of parentification. The image may reflect this as the cat (S)

Administering and Scoring the SDT

Suppose you took a few sips of a soda, then a few more, and more, until your glass was empty. Can you draw lines in the glasses to show how the soda would look if you gradually drank it all?

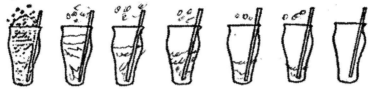

5

Suppose you tilted a bottle half filled with water. Can you draw lines in the bottles to show how the water would look?

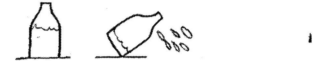

1

Suppose you put the house on the spot marked x. Can you draw the way it would look?

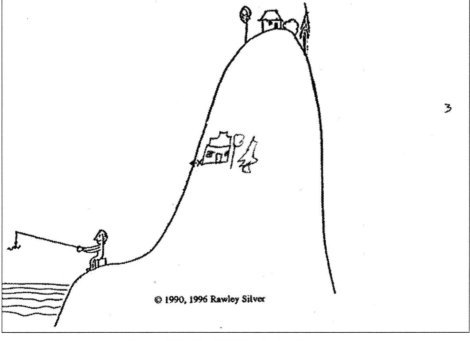

© 1990, 1996 Rawley Silver

3

Figure 10.1. S's SDT Predictive Drawing.

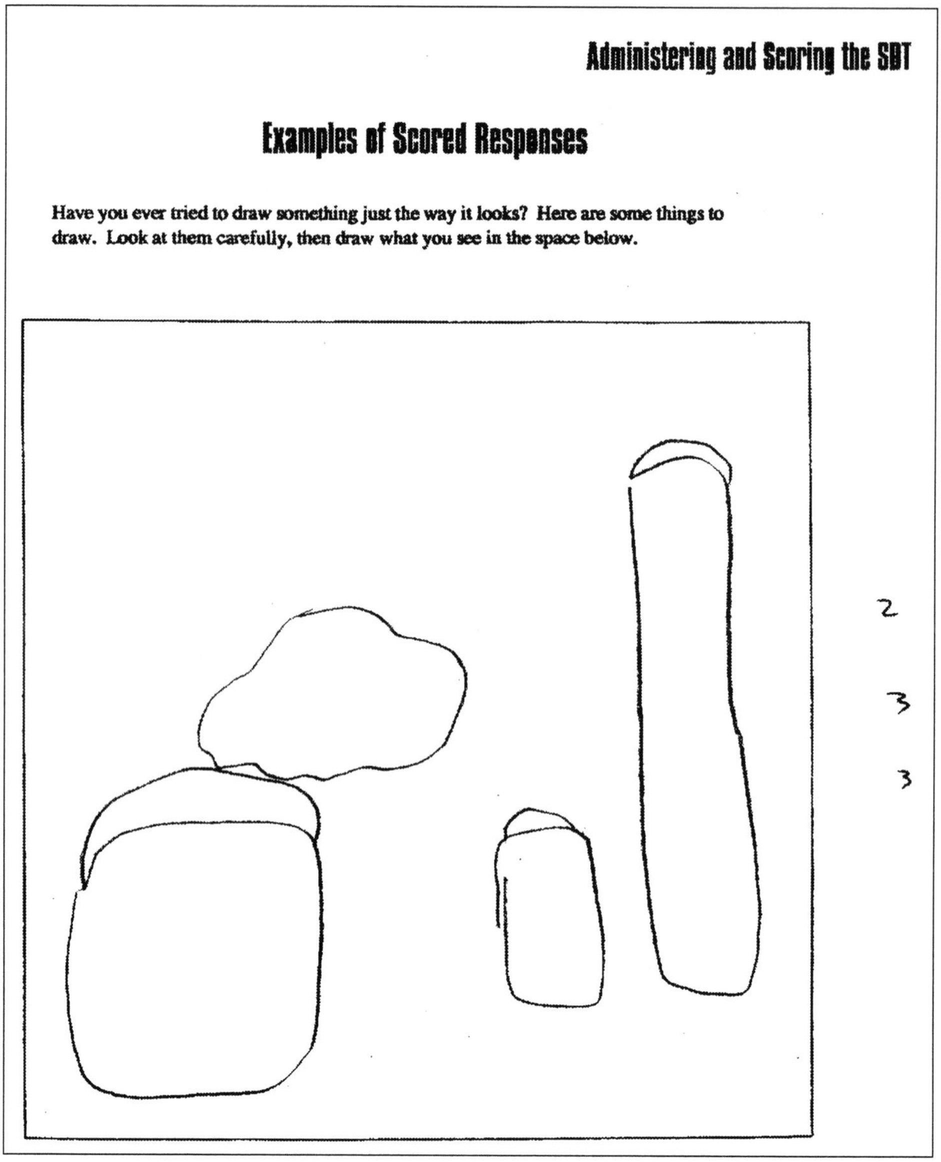
Administering and Scoring the SDT
Examples of Scored Responses
Have you ever tried to draw something just the way it looks? Here are some things to draw. Look at them carefully, then draw what you see in the space below.
2
3
3

Figure 10.2. S's SDT Drawing From Observation.

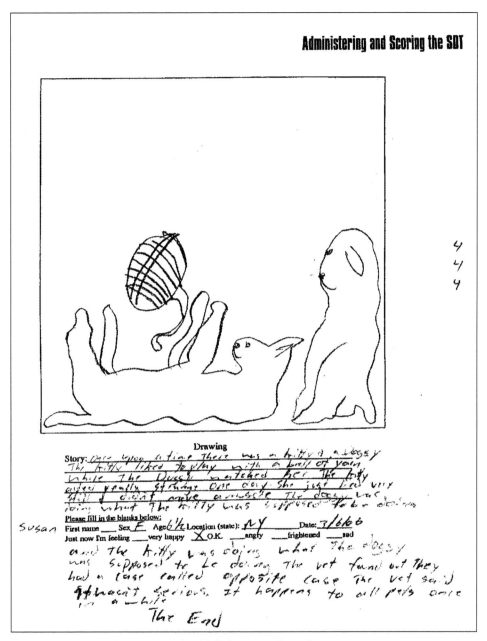

Figure 10.3. S's SDT Drawing From Imagination.

is trying to balance the ball (health, school, family, etc.) and the dog (Mom) is just watching; whereas, the mother should be doing the balancing and the child should be observing (a case of opposite case).

Identified Patient: Nathan

CA: 26.9

DOB: April 5, 1979

Testing Date: April 2, 2006

Administrant: Sarah L. Eksten

Assessments Administered: ATDA, KFD, SDT

See Chapters 1, 2, and 8 for further examples regarding Nathan.

Refer to Appendix A for Genogram, Timeline, Behavioral Observations, and Psychosocial Indicators.

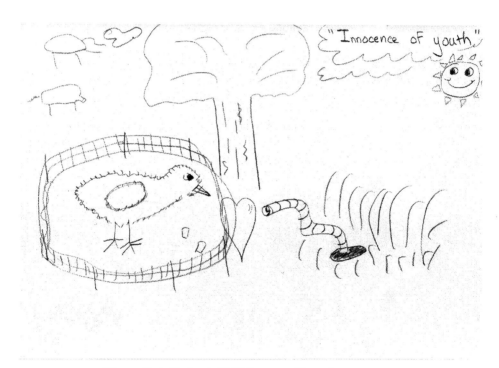

Figure 10.4. Nathan's SDT Drawing From Imagination.

Nathan completed the SDT (Silver, 2002), indicating he was feeling "O.K." before he began the art piece. He titled his work "Innocence of youth." Nathan described the story pertaining to his picture: "It is about the two young animals in the picture: the chick and the worm. They don't know they are suppose to be enemies, so they become friends and fall in love." Nathan goes on to say that the two animals were not "pre-conditioned" to be enemies; therefore, this allowed them to become friends. The writer asked if the two animals represented anyone in his life; however, Nathan said they did not. The administrant asked the client if the animals' parents were in their lives. Nathan responded by saying that, yes, they were around and present; however, the picture represented one instance in the animals' lives which the parents were not there for. Tables 1 and 2 depict the scores provided by the writer to assess for the emotional content of the principle subjects and environment of the drawing as well as for evaluating cognitive and creative skills through a response drawing, respectively (Silver, 2002). From reviewing the scores assigned by the writer, it can be concluded that Nathan may be aware of his emotions and can freely express them through art. Also, he may be approximately average with his cognitive or creative skills.

In addition to the basic theme of the picture, further details may explain other characteristics about the client. The choice of the chick is essentially an expression of a wish to escape from a stressful and unyielding situation (Levy & Levy, 1958). However, this bird looks like it is unable to fly, reinforcing the idea that Nathan may be unable to get away from the situation. The tree drawn with two lines for a trunk and a looped crown is a good indicator that Nathan may be impulsive (Oster & Crone, 2004). There was also no visible groundline, which may suggest that he is vulnerable to stress or unstable (Oster & Crone, 2004). Moreover, there were no roots on the trees, which may suggest repressed emotions (Oster & Crone, 2004). There is a sun included, although personified, that may display a positive outlook on life.

Recommendations and Conclusions

By comparing all three assessments, overall conclusions can be determined regarding Nathan's characteristics. The fact that Nathan used pencil for all drawings, even when he was able to use coloring media, may conclude that Nathan is afraid to explore any emotions surrounding the drawings he completed since color is known to extract feelings and emotions. In addition, all the drawings, for the most part, lacked symmetry, indicating that Nathan may have inadequate feelings of security in his emotional life (Hammer, 1958). This challenges the score Nathan obtained in the Stimulus Drawing that indicated he may be aware of his emotions and can freely express them through art. All the drawings contained straightline strokes, which may be present in individuals who tend to be assertive (Hammer, 1958). The drawings of himself in each picture lacked hands, possibly signifying feelings of trouble or inadequacy (Oster & Crone, 2004). In the drawings that contained trees, most of them had two lines for a trunk and a looped crown, possibly displaying impulsive characteristics (Oster & Crone, 2004). All the trees in the pictures either had no or a very minimal root system, which may insinuate that Nathan represses some of his emotions (Oster & Crone, 2004). Each picture was lacking a definite groundline, which could imply that Nathan is vulnerable to stress or that he is unstable (Oster & Crone, 2004). Both the ATDA (see Chapter 2) and SDT uncovered possible unconscious thoughts of escape from some situation in his life.

From reviewing the drawings, the writer concluded that Nathan falls between Lowenfeld and Brittain's Schematic Stage (7–9 years) and Gang Age (9–12 years) (Horovitz, 2002). The drawings were more conceptual rather than perceptual. They also had a bold, direct representation with the organization of objects being mostly two-dimensional and there being little overlap; however, there was some awareness to detail. In addition, Nathan expressed the self-consciousness of his drawings. There still seemed to be no understanding of shade and shadow; although, there was less exaggeration of body parts and more stiffness of figures.

The administrant suggests that although there seemed to be no significant indications of problems that were a cause for concern from reviewing these three assessments, she feels that Nathan may still benefit from occasional Art Therapy to release any stress he may be encountering. It may also be beneficial in that it may help him become more in touch with his feelings and emotions, and he may learn ways of expressing them. Art Therapy can also be used as an opportunity to sort out any feelings of trouble or inadequacy that may be occurring, or to explore his impulsivity.

Table 1
Emotional Content of Principle Subjects and Environments

Principle Subjects

6 points – moderately positive, for example, subjects who are effective, strong, or fortunate

Environment

7 points – strongly positive, for example, loving or deeply gratifying relationships

(Silver, 2002)

Table 2
Cognitive and Creative Skills

Content (Ability to select)

2 points – between perceptual level and functional level

Form (Ability to Combine)

3 points – subjects are related along a base-line, real or implied

Creativity (Ability to Represent)

3 points – changes or elaborates on SDs or stereotypes

(Silver, 2002)

Identified Patient: Pam

DOB: August, 1954

CA: 52

Testing Dates: September 27, 2006; March 21, 2007; March 28, 2007

Administrant: Julie Riley

Assessments Administered: BATA, FSA, SDT

See Chapters 3 and 6 for further examples regarding Pam.

Predictive Drawing	5	
Drawing From Observation	9	
Drawing From Imagination	6	[emotional content 3; self image 3]
Total	20	

Pam received a score of 20 out of a possible 45. She received a zero for both the predicting a sequence and predicting verticality due to the lack of any soda representation and the drawing of the house within the mountain. Pam also showed significant impairment in representing depth for the Drawing from Observation subtest obtaining a score of 1. In patients with brain injuries, "executive functioning, reasoning, problem-solving abilities, and field-neglect problems . . . became evident if the patient drew closer to one side of the page or the other" (Silver, 2002, p. 181). This phenomenon can be seen in Pam's Drawing from the Imagination Subtest. During administration of the Silver Drawing Test, Pam presented high levels of discomfort and agitation. Overly concerned with the aspect of testing, she repeatedly asked the administrant if it was "going to be graded." Pam had been tested many times in the 36 years since the onset of her TBI; this assessment possibly triggered anxieties due to previous association with tests administered.

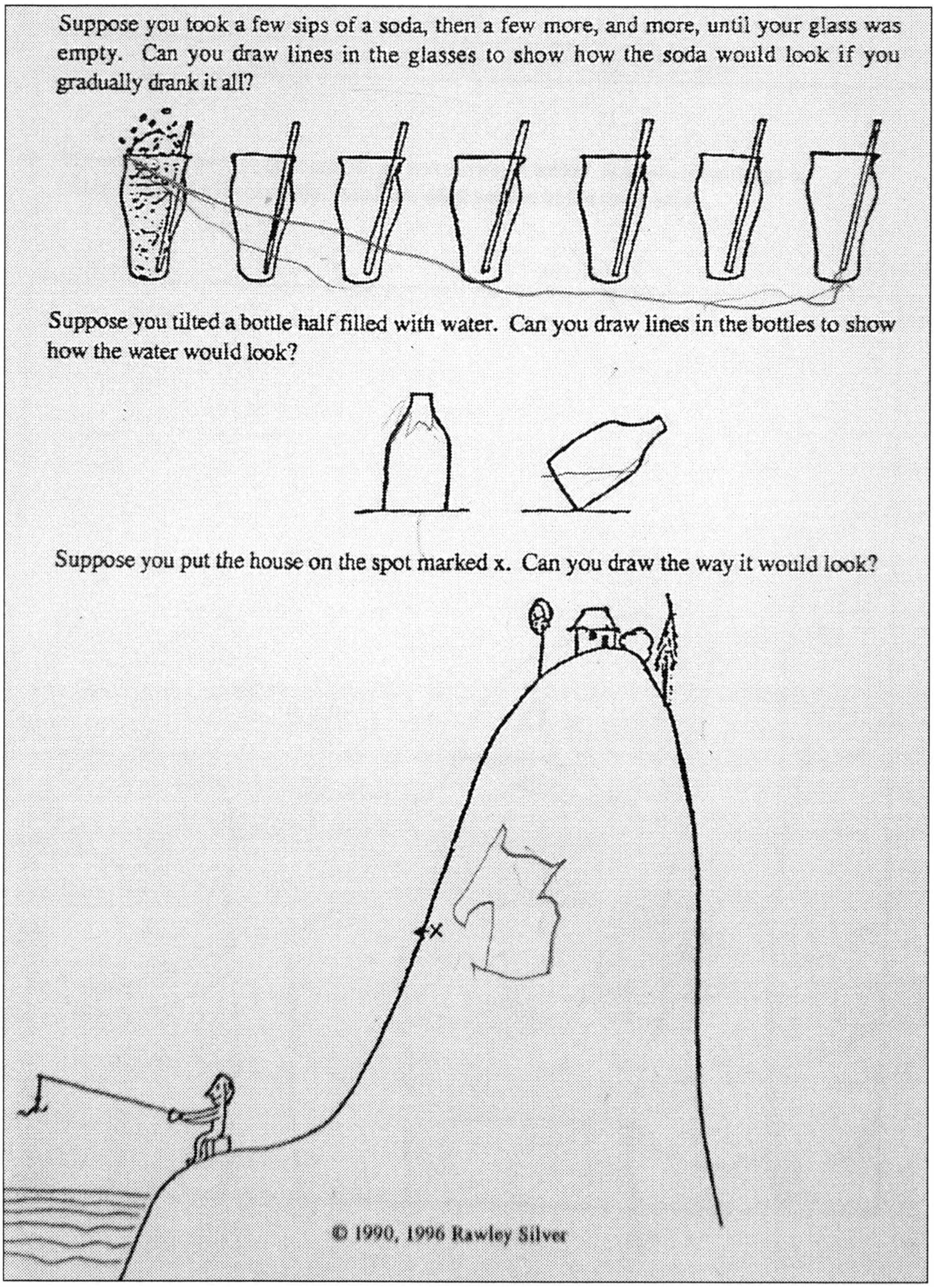
Suppose you took a few sips of a soda, then a few more, and more, until your glass was empty. Can you draw lines in the glasses to show how the soda would look if you gradually drank it all?
Suppose you tilted a bottle half filled with water. Can you draw lines in the bottles to show how the water would look?
Suppose you put the house on the spot marked x. Can you draw the way it would look?
x
© 1990, 1996 Rawley Silver

Figure 10.5. Pam's SDT Predictive Drawing.

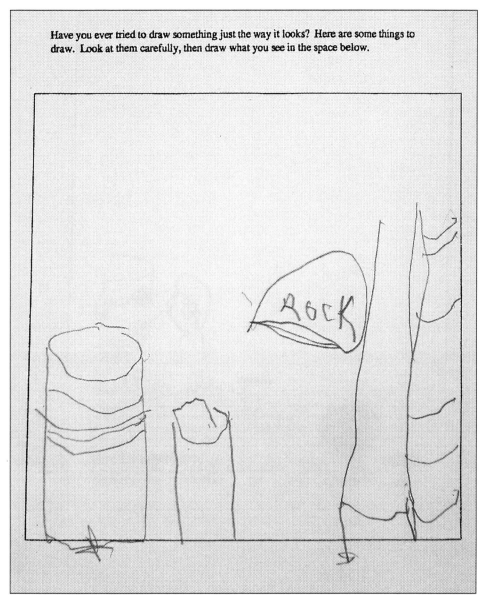

Have you ever tried to draw something just the way it looks? Here are some things to draw. Look at them carefully, then draw what you see in the space below.

Figure 10.6. Pam's SDT Drawing From Observation.

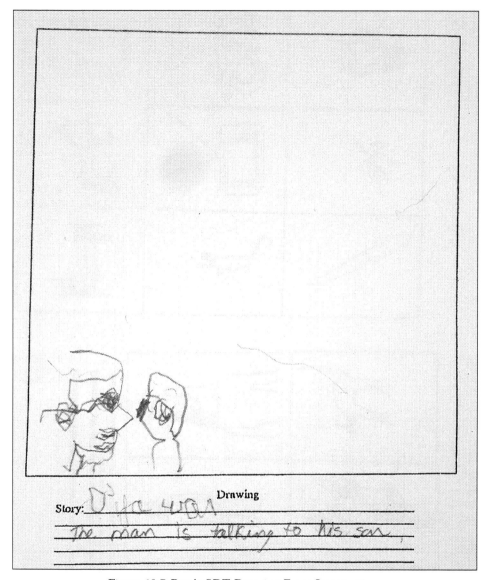

Figure 10.7. Pam's SDT Drawing From Imagination.

Chapter 11

FROM AFRICA TO AMERICA: ART ASSESSMENTS WITH A REFUGEE IN RESETTLEMENT

In this example below, James (Jim) Albertson conducted one of the most thorough assessments that ever passed before Horovitz in her year-long assessment class. Jim had been privy to working with this client throughout the semester and thus was able to draw significant conclusions based on the IP's (Alexander) genogram, timeline, and cultural diversity. Six art-based assessments were conducted with an adult refugee from Burundi, Africa currently in his eighth month of resettlement in Rochester, NY. Jim's excellent synopsis of this unusual case is presented below.

Introduction

Assessing the mental health of refugees in resettlement is a complex process that is often convoluted by language and intercultural barriers (Misra, Connolly, & Majeed, 2006; Savin, Seymour, Littleford, & Giese, 2005). Given traditional and cultural norms, combined with the stress created by resettlement itself, refugees may find it difficult to create a verbal narrative about their past experiences and current emotional state. For this reason, using the creative arts as a modality to assess the mental health of refugees in resettlement could prove useful. Art therapy assessments can provide a therapist with a means of gathering important clues into the emotional state and cognitive levels of clients in a nonthreatening way. Art therapists often use assessments to determine client strengths and problem areas, to observe the client's reaction to a variety of media, and to discover ways in which the client goes about completing art tasks (Malchiodi, 2003). In addition, these same assessments can provide information to determine the client's overall suitability for art therapy treatment (Malchiodi, 2003). The

177

following paper describes a total of six art-based assessments with an adult refugee from Burundi, Africa currently in his eighth month of resettlement in Rochester, NY. The information provided herein illustrates the application of these assessments and highlights important considerations when working in an intercultural context.

CASE STUDY

Identified Patient: Alexander

CA: 20.4

DOB: December 23, 1987

Administrant: Jim Albertson

Assessments Administered: Cognitive Art Therapy Assessment (CATA)
House-Tree-Person (HTP)
Kinetic Family Drawing (KFD)
Silver Drawing Test (SDT)
Belief Art Therapy Assessment (BATA)
Person Picking an Apple from a Tree (PPAT)

Psychosocial Indicators

Alexander is a 20-year-old Refugee from Burundi, Africa who immigrated to the United States in September of 2006 after living for 12 years at a Refugee camp in Western Tanzania (see Figure 11.14). At the time of resettlement, Alexander, accompanied by his younger brother (age 18), sister (age 17), and nephew (age 3), joined his maternal uncle who had resettled in Rochester, NY after being granted Refugee status three years earlier. Currently, he resides in a three-bedroom apartment in the city with his younger brother and fellow Burundian refugee (age 21). His sister and nephew live in an adjoining apartment with their uncle, aunt, and two children. When reflecting on his relationships with his siblings and extended family, Alexander acknowledged that he was close to both his brother and sister, but expressed some conflict when discussing rapport with his uncle who, in January of this year, was accused of impregnating a 12-year-old refugee (also from Burundi) and was put in jail. As a result of his uncle's incarceration, Alexander has had to take on a considerable amount of responsibility for his brother, sister, and nephew as their legal guardian. When asked about his parents, he stated that he never knew his father and indicated that his mother had died in Burundi from an illness when he was just five years old.

Alexander is currently at a sixth grade level of education, is employed at a local Laundromat, and receives financial support from Social Services. Over the past five months he has been attending English classes offered by the Rochester City School System in preparation for GED classes. Teachers at the school recently expressed concern for Alexander, stating that he has been demonstrating signs of depression and social withdrawal.

Behavioral Observations

Initially, Alexander presented as a somewhat timid Black African man who openly demonstrated lack of self-confidence through his nonverbal communication. Physically, he is a short and thin, dark skinned and looks younger than his actual age. At the first meeting, he was reserved and quiet, presented with closed body language, and was unwilling to make eye contact with this administrant. Taking this into consideration, this writer chose to disclose relevant personal information about his seven years of experience living and working in West Africa. After self-disclosure, the interpersonal dynamic changed immediately. Alexander began to interact with the administrant with a heightened level of trust and agreed to participate in the assessments. Over the course of several meetings, he became increasingly more comfortable, was extremely cooperative, and willing to participate in each art directive. Despite communication in dislike for his artwork, Alexander appeared to receive much pleasure from working with the art materials.

Assessment Results

Cognitive Art Therapy Assessment (CATA)

The first assessment that was administered was the Cognitive Art Therapy Assessment (Horovitz-Darby, 1988). This assessment offers open-ended creative activities with pencil, paint, and clay (Horovitz-Darby, 1988), and seemed like an appropriate starting point for this subject when considering the intercultural context. Not only would it elicit specific kinds of behavior with each of the three materials, it would also provide the administrant with important indicators regarding the subject's familiarity and ability to engage with the art materials for subsequent assessments.

First, the administrant explained to Alexander that he had the choice to draw, paint, and make whatever he wanted from clay, and asked, "With which medium would you like to start?" Though he initially was drawn to the clay, Alexander decided to begin with the pencil drawing because it was "the most difficult."

Pencil Response

For this subtest, Alexander used a pencil to begin drawing what appeared to be a vehicle. After almost 10 minutes, he then erased the image completely and carefully drew a knife and an apple instead. Both objects were drawn in correct proportion to one another and their positioning on the page suggested an implied baseline. When asked why he had erased the initial drawing, Alexander indicated that his first attempt was too difficult and would take him too long to finish. While the erasure of the drawing itself is suggestive of anxiety, when coupled with his attention to the quality of the artwork, it could imply his desire to please the administrat or his need to control his environment (Burns & Kaufman, 1972).

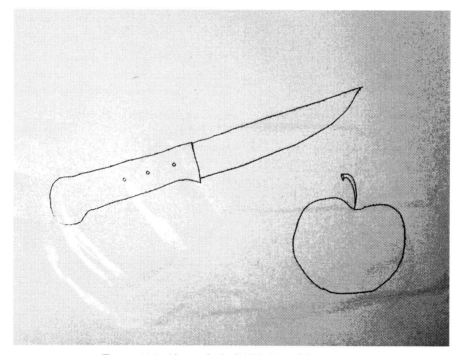

Figure 11.1. Alexander's CATA Pencil Response.

When asked about the final image (see Figure 11.1), Alexander explained that, "The knife is used to cut the apple so that you can eat it." Taking this into consideration, one could postulate that he is struggling with nurturance issues and/or may be harboring some anger about his imposed role as provider for his brother, sister, and nephew.

Painting Response

For the second subtest, Alexander chose to paint. Prior to starting, he explained that he has painted before, but was not familiar with using this particular kind of paint. As anticipated, Alexander demonstrated little knowledge about mixing colors. As a result, this writer showed him how to mix the color green and explained that other colors, when mixed together, would also create new colors. Excited, Alexander quickly grabbed a pencil and paper and wrote down which colors to mix to get orange, purple, green, and light blue. When creating his image, Alexander carefully mixed colors and applied them to the paper with broad strokes. Once the entire surface had been covered, he set down the paint brushes and said he was finished. When describing his image (Figure 11.2), Alexander indicated that this was not a painting of anything in particular and explained that he was just "getting to know how to paint." While his painting was not representational, he was able to effectively engage with the materials to create a well-balanced composition between warm and cool colors. Furthermore, he demonstrated incredible control with the paint, and appeared pleased with his efforts to mix the paint.

Figure 11.2. Alexander's CATA Paint Response.
(For color version, see Plate 28, p. 122.)

Clay Response

For his final subtest, the clay component, Alexander created two remarkable vessels. The first (Figure 11.3a), which took approximately 15 minutes to create, resembled a typical drinking mug that could be found anywhere. The second piece (Figure 11.3b), however, required roughly 25 minutes to create and was described as a "traditional African pot – the kind used for cooking." During the process, this writer noted Alexander's observable familiarity with the materials and asked if he had ever worked with clay before. He then explained how as a child he used to make small animals and airplanes out of clay. He and his friends would bake the clay figures in the sun and then play with them once they were hard. As he recounted the story, Alexander smiled, suggesting that this was a fond memory for him.

When looking at the final products, Alexander was clearly able to attain sculptural form. In both instances, he demonstrated a keen knowledge of the materials and remained engaged with no regression. During the 40 minutes it took to complete this subtest, Alexander was invested in his artwork and when finished, he expressed satisfaction with his efforts. Important to note is the nurturance symbolism of both vessels, which reinforces the pencil subtest as indicative of a possible struggle with nurturance issues.

Overall, Alexander responded well to all three mediums and produced a successful product in each instance. Furthermore, demonstrating both technical skill and control, he was able to didactically engage with the materials – particularly when mixing paint. This suggests that Alexander has the capacity to use the art materials as a modality for artistic expression and, developmentally, would place his artwork within the adult stage/artistic stage (Horovitz, 2002).

House-Tree-Person (HTP)

Alexander's achromatic HTP generated qualities that were consistent in all three drawings. First, Alexander lightly sketched out each image before reinforcing the lines with heavier strokes. While heavy consistent strokes and firm lines are usually indicative of a great deal of drive and ambition (Hammer, 1958), when drawn in this manner, they could indicate a superficial veneer of confidence and boldness (Hammer, 1958). In addition, each image was drawn centered on the page – typical in subjects that display a high degree of self-direction and emotional behavior (Hammer, 1958).

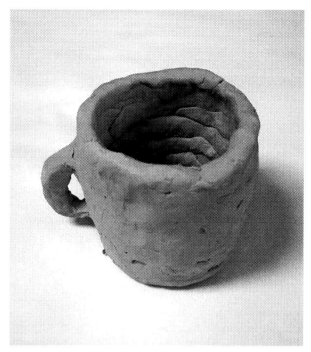

Figure 11.3a. Alexander's CATA Clay Response #1.

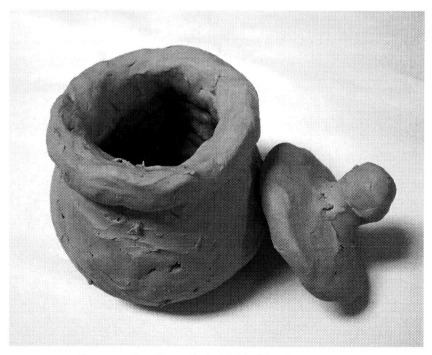

Figure 11.3b. Alexander's CATA Clay Response #2.

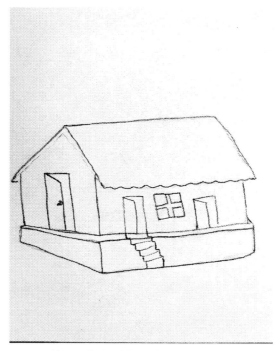

Figure 11.4. Alexander's HTP Achromatic House Response.

House

The house drawing has been found to arouse associations concerning home life and interfamilial relationships (Hammer, 1958). Alexander's depiction of a house (Figure 11.4), which he identified as "a house in Africa," contains several notable characteristics. First, while the house is structurally sound, suggesting a higher degree of ego-strength (Hammer, 1958), there is clearly no groundline, leaving the house floating in the center of the page. According to Hammer (1958), this can be indicative of a fragile contact with reality and suggests that Alexander's strong sense of ego is not grounded. This could also reflect Alexander's current struggle with assimilating into American culture and related feelings of inadequacy.

Equally important is the inclusion of three separate doors on his house. While this is typical in traditional African structures, each door could represent each of the three siblings. The fact that all three doors are open suggests that there is a strong need to receive warmth from the outside world (Oster & Crone, 2004). Furthermore, one of the doors was drawn significantly larger than the other two. Hammer (1958) states that overly large doors are drawn by those individuals who give other clinical evidence of being overly-dependent upon others.

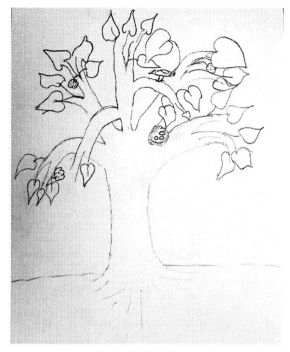

Figure 11.5. Alexander's HTP Achromatic Tree Response.

In addition to these apparent characteristics, one can also see that there is no chimney in his drawing. According to Oster and Crone (2004), it is possible that this implies a lack in psychological warm and could also indicate conflicts with significant male figures. While this seems congruent to Alexander's lack of a father figure and current relationship with his uncle, it is import to note that houses in contemporary African culture do not normally include a chimney.

Tree

In his tree response (Figure 11.5), Alexander's feelings of inadequacy and vulnerability to stress are again illustrated by the faint groundline (Oster & Crone, 2004). This is similar to the line employed to draw the trunk of the tree, which could also indicate feelings of impending personality collapse or loss of identity (Hammer, 1958). When considering the complex implications of the resettlement process on identity, this makes sense. However, despite these feelings, Alexander's branches on his tree are reaching out. This suggests that he does have the resources needed to seek satisfaction from the environment (Hammer, 1958).

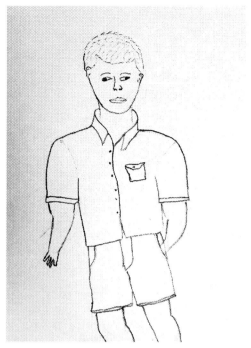

Figure 11.6. Alexander's HTP Achromatic Person Response.

Other notable characteristics in the tree drawing include his emphasis on the crown of the tree, signifying emotional inhibition (Oster & Crone, 2004), and the inclusion of the bird's nest with three eggs. Again, the number of the eggs could represent the three siblings and their need for nurturance.

Person

For his person, Alexander drew what he described as "any man" and made it clear to this writer that he was neither "American or African." This suggests Alexander could be struggling with important identity issues that were also evident in his tree response. When looking at the final image (Figure 11.6), one can see that the head is slightly enlarged, which has been said to be a sign of a preoccupation with fantasy life or a focus on mental life (Oster & Crone, 2004). Again, this may well be a reflection of Alexander's need for psychological warmth that was also seen in the house subtest. The omission of the feet and depiction of small hands indicates that he could be feeling a lack of independence/interpersonal mobility, as well as the inability to control or manipulate his environment (Oster & Crone, 2004).

When looking at the finer details of the drawing, one can see that Alexander's person's eyes are crossed. For refugees who find themselves in resettlement after being displaced by civil war and conflict, the future is often unclear. Perhaps the crossed eyes represent Alexander's lack of vision for his own future. Other interesting characteristics in the person drawing include the large shoulders, indicative of a preoccupation with perceived need for strength (Oster & Crone, 2004), and his depiction of one hand in the pocket of his shorts, suggesting troubled feelings or feelings of inadequacy.

Silver Drawing Test (SDT)

The Silver Drawing Test is an art-based assessment that has both cognitive and emotional components and is made up of three subtests: Drawing from Imagination, Predictive Drawing, and Drawing from Observation. Below are Alexander's scores for each.

Predictive Drawing: 13
Drawing from Observation: 15
Drawing from Imagination: 13

For the first subtest (Figure 11.7), Alexander scored extremely well on predictive elements of sequences and horizontality, however struggled with predicting verticality. While the house was drawn with vertical orientation, it lacked support and was not actually touching the mountain. For this reason, it received a score of three out of five. In his Drawing from Observation (Figure 11.8), Alexander was able to represent all horizontal, vertical, and depth relations. Because his drawing was so accurate, this writer scored the subtest with a five despite the omission of the layout sheet (normally required to receive a full score).

For the third and final subtest, Alexander was presented with Form A of the stimulus drawings and was given the directive to choose at least two of the drawings and think of a story about these pictures. Once he had his idea, he was instructed to then draw his own picture of something happening between them. Without much hesitation, Alexander selected the cat and the snake from the form. For his drawing (Figure 11.9), he simply copied the stimulus pictures inside the provided space with no embellishment. When he was finished, Alexander wrote the following phrase beneath his picture: "A snake want to eat a cat and a cat was angry and he get the snake."

In ability to select, Alexander's response is a well-organized idea and, when coupled with his statement below the picture, implies more than is visible. Taking this into consideration a score of five seemed most appropriate. When looking at the form of the completed drawing, one can see that the subjects are related to one another on an implied baseline, but do not show depth beyond this perspective. For this reason, Alexander scored a three out of five on his ability to combine. In ability to represent, Alexander received a score of five, as his drawing was both expressive and highly suggestive.

188

The Art Therapists' Primer

Administering and Scoring the SDT

Suppose you took a few sips of a soda, then a few more, and more, until your glass was empty. Can you draw lines in the glasses to show how the soda would look if you gradually drank it all?

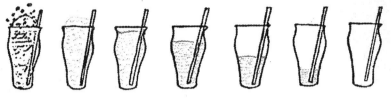

Suppose you tilted a bottle half filled with water. Can you draw lines in the bottles to show how the water would look?

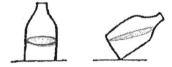

Suppose you put the house on the spot marked x. Can you draw the way it would look?

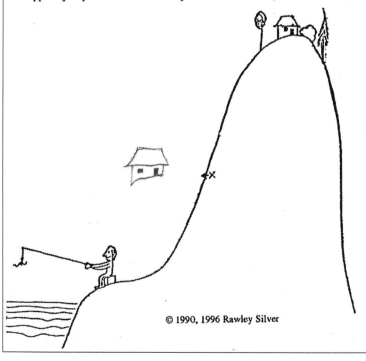

© 1990, 1996 Rawley Silver

Figure 11.7. Alexander's SDT Predictive Drawing.

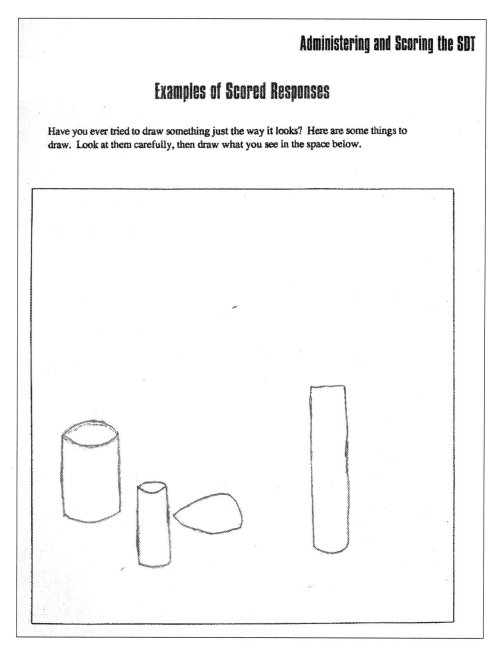

Administering and Scoring the SDT

Examples of Scored Responses

Have you ever tried to draw something just the way it looks? Here are some things to draw. Look at them carefully, then draw what you see in the space below.

Figure 11.8. Alexander's SDT Drawing From Observation.

In emotional content, the theme of Alexander's drawing is strongly negative and received a score of one. The depiction of the cat and snake elicit both fear and aggression and suggest a life-threatening relationship. For self

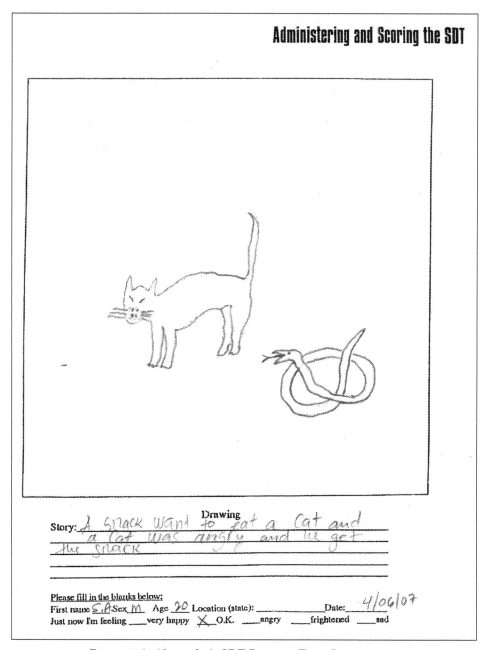

Figure 11.9. Alexander's SDT Drawing From Imagination.

image, Alexander may have identified with the feelings that either the cat or the snake possessed, but no direct correlation was made. For this reason a score of 3 was given.

Overall, Alexander scored very well on all three subtests, with a final score of 41 out of 45. This suggests that cognitively he is functioning quite well and has a high aptitude for learning.

Kinetic Family Drawing (KFD)

Burns and Kaufman (1972) suggest the Kinetic-Family Drawing often reflects primary disturbances much more quickly and adequately than interviews or other probing techniques administered by clinicians. This premise holds true for Alexander's KFD results (Figure 11.10).

In response to the directive, draw yourself and your family doing something, Alexander produced a drawing of his brother "cutting" (sawing) a board into two halves. While technically this drawing was quite impressive, the response itself is rather unusual. When considering the concept of "family" in the context of African culture, where people identify themselves in relation to the family system rather than as an individual, one would expect to see representation of both immediate and extended family members. Alexander's decision to exclude everyone but his brother from his drawing could indicate conflict regarding his relationships with other family members

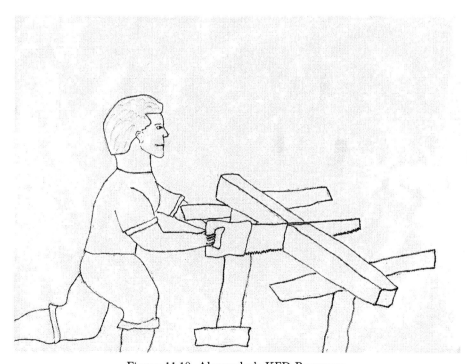

Figure 11.10. Alexander's KFD Response.

and/or confusion about his own role within the family system (Burns & Kaufman, 1972). This could be a result of ambivalent feelings towards his uncle, as well as his responsibility as legal guardian of his siblings and nephew.

When examining the content of the drawing itself, there are several elements that need to be noted. First, Alexander drew his brother sawing a plank-like board, which could be compared to a log. Burns and Kaufman (1972) explain that logs are often associated with hyper-masculinity or masculine striving. The fact that Alexander has depicted his brother sawing this log in half could indicate feelings of castration and a lack of virility. In addition, the two halves of the board could represent his struggle with the duality of holding on to his African culture/tradition and, at the same time, assimilating into western society.

When looking at the figure itself, one can see that Alexander omitted his brother's feet. This is similar to his person drawing (see Figure 11.6) in the HTP Assessment and again indicates a lack of independence (Oster & Crone, 2004). Also important, is the use of the saw as an extension of the hand/arm which Burns and Kaufman (1972) postulate could suggest the ability to better control his environment. Since his brother was allowed to attend high school upon arrival to the United States and he was not, Alexander may perceive him as having more control over his environment.

Person Picking an Apple from a Tree (PPAT)

In response to the directive, "Draw a person picking an apple from a tree," Alexander drew a picture of an "American man" kneeling on the ground to pick the apple (Figure 11.11). Both the position of the man and his size in proportion to the tree suggest that nurturance and sustenance are easily attainable for Americans. This could reflect Alexander's own feelings of inadequacy stemming from the inability to meet his needs as a refugee in resettlement. When looking further at the content of the drawing, one can see that the tree itself is drawn with two-dimensional branches that are unclosed. According to Hammer (1958), this could indicate a feeling of little control over the expression of one's impulses. In addition, the branches in the tree also appear broken or cut-off. This has been said to suggest feelings of being traumatized and/or castrated on both the psychosocial level (feelings of inadequacy, helplessness, and enforced passivity) and psychosexual level (lack of virility) (Hammer, 1958).

Using the Formal Art Therapy Scale (FEATS) one can begin to assess the formal elements and characteristics of drawings (Gantt & Tabone, 1998). When rated on all 14 scales, Alexander received a total score of 53 out of 70. Despite not using the entire page, Alexander did create a fairly integrated

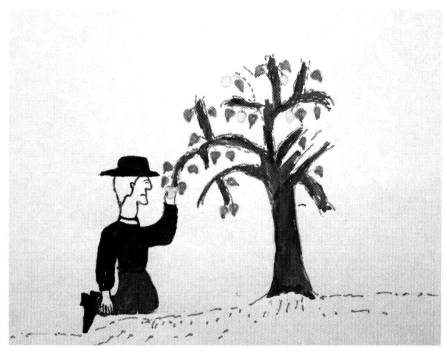

Figure 11.11. Alexander's PPAT Response. (For color version, see Plate 29, p. 123.)

composition that was recognizable and somewhat complex; and he used appropriate colors to both outline and fill in some, but not all, of the forms and objects in the drawing. While several of the scales do indicate signs of mild depression, overall, most are suggestive of a nonpatient response.

Belief Art Therapy Assessment (BATA)

The final assessment that was administered was the Belief Art Therapy Assessment (Horovitz, 2002). This writer began by asking Alexander a series of questions provided in the history-taking portion of the BATA as outlined in *Spiritual Art Therapy: An Alternate Path* (Horovitz, 2002). Given the inter-cultural context and some language limitations, several questions were altered in order to obtain appropriate information. When asked about his religious affiliation, Alexander indicated that he was currently a Christian. However, he quickly added that he had been raised as a Muslim and only converted to Catholicism in 2004 while living in the Refugee camp in Tanzania. When asked why he changed his belief, Alexander stated that when he was a Muslim his "heart was not good." After reading the Bible and comparing it to the Qur'an, he decided that Christianity was better for him and said it made his "heart feel better." It is important to note here that several of Alexander's Uncles, including the one living in Rochester, were opposed to his religious conversion. For that reason, he did not become a Christian until these uncles had left the Refuge camp in 2004. In regards to his current practices, Alexander indicated that he is attending a Christian church regularly but does not actively participate outside of the weekly service. Before moving on to the art directive, Alexander told this writer that he feels he has a personal relationship with God and it is this relationship that gives him strength and meaning in his life.

This administrant then asked Alexander to use any art materials he liked to draw, paint, or sculpt what God meant to him. In response, Alexander chose to use pencil and paint, and simultaneously drew what God means to him as well as the opposite of God (Figure 11.12). When asked to describe his drawing, Alexander explained that there are two paths: one towards the devil and one towards God. He then expanded on this by saying, "God is a choice" and that ultimately "one wants to be going in the direction of God." This duality is well illustrated with his use of arrows to depict the different paths. When discussing the image further, Alexander stated that going in the right direction is a constant struggle for him. Despite this struggle, he did draw his figure with feet, which suggests that this is one aspect of his life that he does have control over.

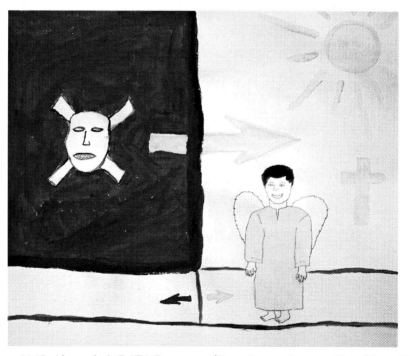

Figure 11.12. Alexander's BATA Response. (For color version, see Plate 30, p. 123.)

When considering the information provided by Alexander regarding his belief and continued struggle with going in the "right direction," this writer placed him in Stage 4 of Spiritual Development according to James Fowler. According to Horovitz (2002), Fowler states that this stage typically occurs in young adulthood and is identified by unavoidable tensions regarding accountability and responsibility for one's lifestyle, commitments, attitudes, and beliefs.

Overall Developmental Level of the Artwork

- Cognitive Art Therapy Assessment (CATA): Adult stage/artistic stage (Horovitz, 2002)
- House-Tree-Person (HTP)/Kinetic Family Drawing (KFD)/Person Picking an Apple from a Tree (PPAT): Pseudo-Naturalistic Stage, 12–14 years as defined by Lowenfeld and Brittain.
- Belief Art Therapy Assessment (BATA): Pseudo-Naturalistic Stage, 12–14 years as defined by Lowenfeld and Brittain.

Conclusions and Recommendations

In all six assessments, Alexander was successful in his attempts at formed expression and produced artwork with evocative power and consistency. His ability to engage and learn from the materials, and extract pleasure from each product suggests normal cognitive and emotional development. When reflecting on both the artwork that he produced, and his psychosocial and behavioral indicators, one can postulate that Alexander is struggling with ambivalent feelings about his role as provider juxtaposed by his own needs for nurturance. Also, rather than exhibit signs of pathological depression, Alexander seems to be suffering from feelings of helplessness (little control over his environment), inadequacy, and forced passivity.

Given his ability and willingness to engage with the art materials, Alexander would benefit from individual art therapy as a means of expressing his struggle to adapt to American society and also confront the dualities that have surfaced in his artwork regarding his identity. Furthermore, given his response to the Belief Art Therapy Assessment, it seems logical to incorporate a spiritual component from the onset of treatment.

Alexander's Genogram Timeline: History

1987 – Alexander is born in Burundi.

1989 – Brother is born.

1990 – Sister is born.

1992 – Mother dies from illness in Burundi at age 45.

1994 – At age 6, Alexander and his siblings are displaced to Tanzania with his maternal uncle as a result of civil war and conflict in Burundi.

2004 – Uncle, his wife, and kids are granted refugee status to the United States and relocate to Rochester, NY. In the same year, his sister (age 14) gives birth to a son in the refugee camp.

2004 – Alexander converts from Islam to Catholicism.

2006 – Alexander, his two siblings, and his nephew are granted asylum in Rochester with their Uncle and immigrate to the United States in September.

2007 – Uncle is accused of impregnating a 12-year-old refugee (also from Burundi) and is put in jail. Alexander becomes the legal guardian of his bother, sister, and her son.

Belief System: Alexander was raised as a Muslim; however, he converted to Christianity (Catholicism) in 2004 while living at the refugee camp in Tanzania. Alexander regularly attends church services.

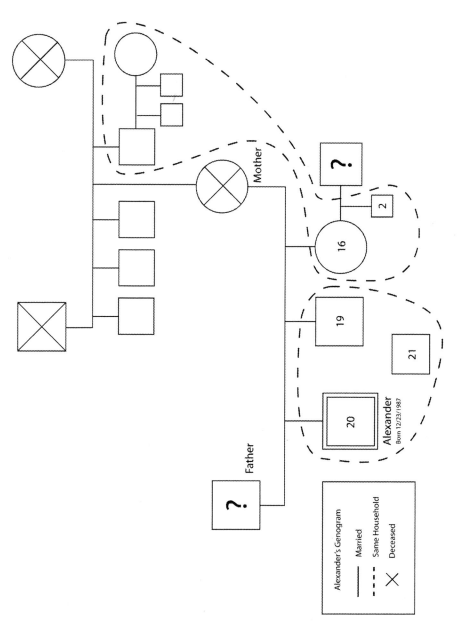

Figure 11.13. Alexander's Genogram.

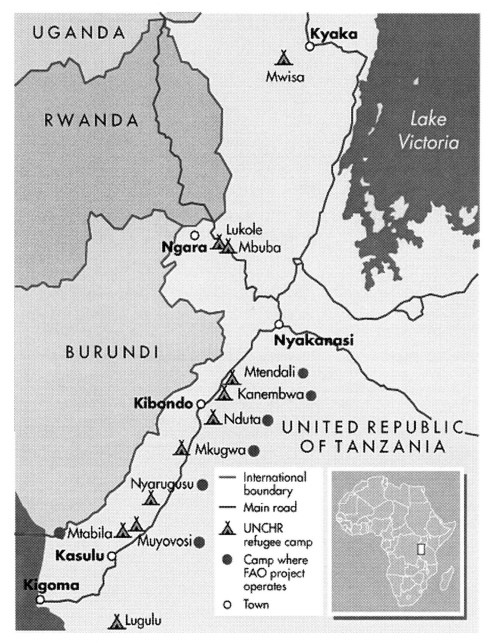

Figure 11.14. Map indicating placement of Refugee Camps
along the Tanzania-Burundi Border.

Chapter 12

ASSESSMENTS, TREATMENT, TERMINATION SUMMARIES AND INTERNET-BASED REFERRALS

Ellen G. Horovitz

In this final chapter, Horovitz presents varying assessments and treatment samples that one might see when working on an interdisciplinary team or as a private practitioner. Abbreviated assessments, a creative arts therapy termination summary, a long-term Art Therapy Termination summary (complete with objectives), and a sample from an Internet-based referral are amongst the highlights of this chapter. These are offered as illustrations of what a practitioner (neophyte or experienced) might bump up against in career and private practice. It is important to note that all of these formats were fashioned by Horovitz at the inception of her career.

In 1980, Horovitz started work in numerous medical settings: residential placements, outpatient treatment, day treatment facilities, and the like. Because her work was conducted in a medical model, she decided to create assessments that dovetailed with other clinical reports. Most importantly, she transliterated her information into medical terminology so that all treatment team members could understand the art therapy assessment process, significant sessions, and objectives and modalities that united with the interdisciplinary treatment team's approach. This was extremely important for several reasons: (a) it placed her on equal footing with social workers, psychologists, psychiatrists, and like mental health workers, and created a platform of respect for her discipline; (b) when the files of clients left her employ and "followed" the client to the next level of care, the records served to inform future practitioners of her work and served as a point of departure for the next creative art therapist (if the client were to receive that level of care); and

(c) her work served as foundation for other creative art therapists and led to her amassing this information in her first *Art Therapy Program Textbook* (which was published in 1995).

This textbook (gingerly referred to as the *Bible* by her students) became a wellspring of not just assessments but also numerous clinical forms for documentation including a legend of abbreviations of clinical and psychiatric terms (used in many of the papers herein and numerous medical settings). That glossary and other pertinent information, such as when to record significant events, are also found in Appendices C thru G of this book. Horovitz's rationale for creating the *Art Therapy Program Textbook* and amassing these forms was to fill a void that had been missing in her own graduate training. Hopefully, these will serve as templates for future practitioners.

Level of Care and Appropriate Treatment

The first sample below is an abbreviated Art Therapy assessment where the client was determined to be *unacceptable* for the level of care offered in Horovitz's outpatient Creative Arts Therapy Clinic at Nazareth College. The biological mother referred the client, DH, to the Creative Arts Therapy Clinic. Horovitz was sought out because of her familiarity with Deafness and fluency in sign language. Nevertheless, it became clear that DH was unsuitable for treatment at this clinic. This was based on not only aggressive and inappropriate behavior, but also lack of medical staffing at the college, necessitated to accept this young man into the level of care available at this college-based outpatient clinic. In this first case, DH refused to use art materials. Through observation, Horovitz was able to engage with this young man and extract the following information.

Art Therapy Diagnostic Assessment

Name: DH

Address:

CA: 18.7

DOB: 2/22/89

Administrant: Dr. Ellen G. Horovitz, ATR-BC, LCAT

Tests: None, DH refused to participate in any art therapy assessments.

Behavioral Observation and Recommendations

DH arrived with his brother, mother, father and speech therapist for his meeting with the art therapist. He seemed very distraught upon arrival, inappropriately touching the clinic supervisor (Ms. Higgins), and initially resisting going into the therapy room with the art therapist.

Initially, his speech therapist insisted and accompanied him into the art therapy clinic while Ms. Higgins met with DH's mother to conduct an intake interview and construct a family genogram. DH presented as several years younger than his biological age of 18 years, 6 months. He presented as a profoundly Deaf, autistic, Caucasian adolescent who wore digital hearing aids to assist him with his hearing loss.

He currently attended speech therapy and indeed his speech/language therapist arrived at the session and suggested coming into the art therapy room in order to both aid DH with this transition as well as assist in translation if necessary. Both she and DH were equipped with an IChat, a device that assisted DH with communication. Nevertheless, in short order, it appeared that the presence of the speech therapist was inhibiting the interview process. As a result, the art therapist asked the speech therapist to wait outside. Both the art therapist, as well as the speech therapist, assured DH that she would be right outside if needed.

After a few minutes, DH warmed up to the art therapist and while he refused to do any artwork, this art therapist was able to successfully communicate in ASL/sign language/voice and engage DH at her computer using the Photo Booth software program on her computer, then IPhoto, and finally printed out images from DH's multiple digital cameras, which he had stashed in his pant pockets.

While the art therapist was able to engage DH using Photo Booth, Photoshop, and IPhoto, it was very clear that DH was disinterested in engaging with the art materials. As well, several times, the art therapist had to redirect DH when he made inappropriate gestures such as attempting to touch the art therapist's face. While it was clear that DH was doing this out of his desire to connect, it was clear that his boundaries regarding appropriate touch were blurred. Moreover, at the session's end, several times, DH had to be redirected by the art therapist not to hit his mother or Ms. Higgins, who was waiting in the hallway.

Conclusion

While it is quite clear that DH could benefit from working with an art therapist whose work encompasses digitally related art media, he was not deemed appropriate for art therapy at the Nazareth College Art Therapy Clinic due to the nature of the clinic confines. DH was also in need of a well-tailored behavioral management art therapy program; unfortunately, because the Art Therapy Clinic is situated on an academic campus, it is not set up to assist DH with such an intensive program, nor is the clinic able to accept DH based on his inappropriate socialization, interaction deficits, and need for medical services.

Nevertheless, it is highly recommended that DH receive art therapy services from an art therapist in private practice within the Western New York and/or Greater Rochester area. Should a referral be desired, this writer would be happy to assist by providing several names of practitioners in that area.

_____   _____

Dr. Ellen G. Horovitz, ATR-BC, LCAT   Date

The above assessment contained pertinent information to aid this family in seeking an appropriate level of treatment for their son. While he might have been appropriate for art therapy in a behaviorally managed care setting, the Creative Arts Therapy clinic was not staffed nor equipped for this treatment or intervention. As a result, the above assessment's prescription was quite clear in its nature and recommendation. It is important to write up assessments that are not only in keeping with information, but that will also serve to safeguard the client and the practitioners. Safety and ethical issues should always be paramount in the practitioner's mind.

Abbreviated Art Therapy Diagnostic Assessment

Name: Scout

BD: 12/18/86

CA: 11.3

Testing Dates: 12/9/97; 12/16/97; 1/12/98; 2/2/98

Test Administered: Cognitive Art Therapy Assessment (CATA) Paint, Clay, and Drawing subtests; Kinetic Family Drawing (KFD)

Genogram

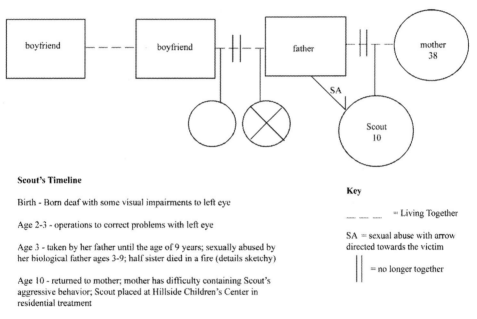

Scout's Timeline

Birth - Born deaf with some visual impairments to left eye

Age 2-3 - operations to correct problems with left eye

Age 3 - taken by her father until the age of 9 years; sexually abused by her biological father ages 3-9; half sister died in a fire (details sketchy)

Age 10 - returned to mother; mother has difficulty containing Scout's aggressive behavior; Scout placed at Hillside Children's Center in residential treatment

Key

_____ ...... _____ = Living Together

SA = sexual abuse with arrow directed towards the victim

‖ = no longer together

Figure 12.1. Scout's Genogram.

Reasons for Referral

Scout was referred because of her inability to engage in verbal communication. It was thought that she would benefit from the nonverbal approach of art therapy. Additionally, while Scout was Deaf, she had not mastered sign language, couldn't communicate well in either PSE (Pigeon Signed English) or ASL (American Sign Language), and primarily used gestures and grunting to delineate her needs.

Behavioral Observations

Scout's responses from the very beginning indicated that she had great difficulty with perceptual pathology. Her responses to all the materials (whether clay, painting, or drawing media) were extremely uncommon. She approached the materials in a type of staccato fashion: her objectivity towards the materials suggested definite organicity and possible neurological impairment. To ascertain whether or not the perceptual pathology precluded developmental gains, the art therapist had suggested a neurological work-up. Scout's developmental delays placed her at the Schematic Stage, age 7–9 years, according to Lowenfeld and Brittain. While this delay was not significantly below her age range, her approach to materials indicated severe difficulty with perception. While reports had indicated previous corrective surgery for her lazy-eye syndrome, her visual acuity still seemed inordinately impaired. Given how visually oriented the Deaf population is, it would be devastating if any of her other senses were taxed. In short, if she were experiencing difficulty with perceptual activity, it would be advantageous to take care of those problems before any further deterioration occurred.

Cognitive Art Therapy Assessment (CATA)

Scout chose to work with the clay medium first and decided to make a mirror frame based on one in the art therapist's office. Interestingly enough, as described above, her approach reflected perceptual pathology and possible visual impairment. While Scout wore corrective eyeglasses and was <u>not</u> wearing them at the time, even with corrective lenses, her responses were the same. The way in which she viewed her work when working was comparable to that of a visually-impaired person (who has pin-hole or tunnel vision) approaching a subject matter: she looked at the material sideways, cocking her head from side-to-side almost inspecting the material in an attempt to understand it. These same features are often witnessed in people that have limited vision – the approach is haptically and kinesthetically oriented as opposed to processing via visual content. Also, her approach when working with the materials reflected an unusual internalization process (e.g., her breathing became heavy as she wedged the clay material) and she appeared to become somewhat exasperated with the actual medium. Nevertheless, her perseverance was quite admirable as she continued to work with the materials. Her method reflected obsessive-compulsive behavior as she repeatedly smoothed the clay until she seemed pleased with the final product. Her final product, a mirror frame, while created because of one that she had seen in the art therapist's office, may also have reflected issues surrounding low self-esteem, self-identity conflicts, and a desire for increased normalcy in her vision.

Her painting responses reflected similar behavior of obsessive-compulsive activity. Repeatedly, Scout requested pink paper for her paintings. Nevertheless, the color of the paper continued to be unrecognizable by the time Scout has finished her project. Predominantly, Scout started off with a meticulous one-fourth inch border completely surrounding the perimeter of the paper. To that she added lines of color and often covered the entire palette with a mixture of purple, red, and blue. The choice of colors may have to do with her past history of physical and sexual abuse, and concomitant desire to control those feelings surrounding the incident. Almost always, Scout covered this work with a muddy brown color, again reflecting a need to obliterate her feelings. Generally, even before the last layer had dried, Scout would scribe her name, as well as the name of her boyfriend, onto the surface. She seemed completely unconcerned with the final effect, which resulted in a muddy picture.

She refused to do the drawing response of the CATA, and again used paints and various media to complete the artwork. In this response, she created a very primitive painting/drawing of a girl with outstretched arms, donning a purple dress and red shoes. The color choice of the clothing and shoes again might have been connected to her previous sexual abuse and her desire to be seductive in fashion. While the arms were outstretched, which suggested Scout's desire to make contact with her environment, the fingers, detailed in mitten-like quality, reflected immaturity. Of interest was the floor-length hair, which served to encapsulate and protect the girl in the picture. Again, this may reflect Scout's need for protection from what she probably has perceived as a rather hostile environment.

All three subsections suggested that Scout was functioning at the upper end of the Schematic Stage of Development, age 7–9 years. These results indicated mild developmental delays.

Kinetic Family Drawing Test (KFD)

Scout was quite resistant to drawing her family and did a light pencil drawing of a house, which she described as her mother's house. She placed her mother and her current boyfriend in one bedroom, and herself and her boyfriend on the other side. These were the only windows detailed on the house, and since they were crafted as second floor windows, clearly the viewer could not witness what was ongoing. Nevertheless, a pathway leading to a large door, complete with doorknob, invited the viewer. So, while bedroom activities appeared to be cloaked, Scout clearly solicited entry.

Once again, developmentally, Scout's work fell into the same category as before: the upper end of the Schematic Stage of Development, age 7–9 years, according to Lowenfeld and Brittain.

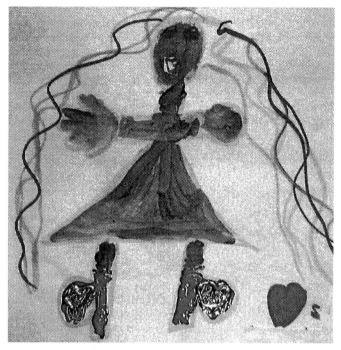

Figure 12.2. Scout's 2nd Painting.

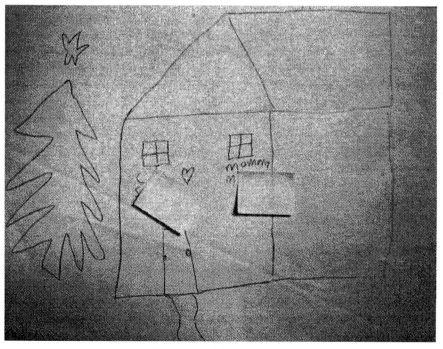

Figure 12.3. Scout's KFD.

Recommendations and Conclusions

As previously mentioned, Scout clearly seemed to display an inordinate amount of perceptual pathology and possible neurological impairment. Given her propensity for navigating her environment through visual processing of information, a complete neurological work-up might uncover more information then currently is on file and is highly recommended. Developmentally, Scout is functioning below age level; although developmentally, she is not terribly off track, Scout functions at approximately the Schematic Stage, age 7–9 years.

While Scout's repertoire includes obsessive-compulsive behavior during making art projects, this "stick-to-it" quality may actually be a strength. She is quite adamant about succeeding in her work and is extremely invested in her artwork, the projects that she makes, and connecting to this worker.

She has already formed a bond to the art therapist (via the testing process) and might actually benefit from sessions that last longer than an hour. She always had to be stopped and if she had her way, she would have stayed at the art therapy studio as long as possible. Clearly, if the art therapist's schedule permitted, it would be recommended to see her at least twice a week. Unfortunately, given this art therapist's current schedule, treatment precludes more than once a week, individual art therapy. The modality, however, will remain flexible to allow for extended sessions. In time, it would be helpful to enfold the mother, half-sister, and mother's current nuclear family (stepmother, boyfriend, and boyfriend's mother) into family art therapy sessions *if* the plan is for Scout to return to home.

The above report reflected the beginning of treatment. For a complete case study see Horovitz (1999). Below is a summation that was placed in Scout's medical file when art therapy was terminated and could be used as a template by other practitioners.

Creative Arts Therapy Termination Template

Creative Arts Therapy Termination Note

Client: Scout

Date of Final Contact: 3/5/99

Therapist: Dr. Ellen G. Horovitz, ATR-BC

Identifying Data

Scout is an attractive and precocious, 11-year-old Caucasian preadolescent female whose demeanor is staccato-like and stunted. While oftentimes she appeared autistic to observers, part of her movements could be attributed to her perceptual pathology and difficulty with vision. While she has a "lazy eye" corrected by surgery and currently eyeglasses, she often examined objects in a rather bizarre manner (e.g., looking at items sideways, jerky head movements in order to "see" an entire object, etc.). As well, Scout was extremely well developed (physically) for someone so young and as a result, she vacillated between seductive behavior with males and infantile behavior with females.

Goals/Objectives

Scout had numerous objectives in order to work towards her goal of returning to home. They were as follows: (a) forming a therapeutic alliance; (b) working on her hygiene issues; (c) focusing on appropriate sexual behavior; (d) communicating more effectively with others; and (e) participating in age-appropriate activities. Scout was able to achieve all of these objectives and had matured considerably since the first meeting of December, 1997. While she experienced a setback when she had intercourse with another client, she continued to do extremely well at her residential cottage and in school.

History of Contacts

There were a total of 33 individual art therapy sessions including one family art therapy session with the mother. The work together was often unorthodox since the focus was on communication and working towards age-appropriate activities. As a result, there was a long period of time (approximately 3–6 months) when Scout and this worker cooked whole meals for the cottage while simultaneously learning how to sew pillows and the like (see sample below).

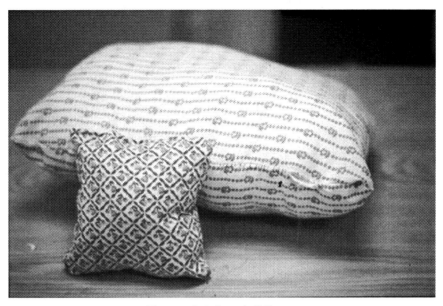

Figure 12.4. Scout's Pillows.

This therapeutic interaction was an attempt to offer appropriate mother-daughter role modeling, something that was vastly missed in her upbringing.

Scout thrived via these activities and changed considerably during the work with the art therapist. When this art therapist initially met Scout, she was an angry, resistant child and at termination she presented as open, gentle, and responsible. While she still has considerable issues around trust, paternal deprivation, and past sexual abuse, she is mostly age-appropriate in her interactions with others. Moreover, she now has considerable command of American Sign Language and communicates more effectively with others.

Major Problems Areas on Referral or At End of Therapy

While Scout continued to struggle with the aforementioned issues (paternal deprivation, need for unconditional nurturance, confusion around appropriate touch and sexual abuse issues), she was beginning to explore some of that work with her movement/dance therapist. Nevertheless, she has expressed a desire to continue in art therapy, should an opening become available. It is highly recommended that she continue individual and/or group art therapy should an opening become available.

_____   _____
Ellen G. Horovitz, Ph.D., ATR-BC   Date
Coordinator of Art Therapy

Assessment of Scout and Creative Arts Termination Summary

When writing about a client, a pseudonym often helps the author relate to that person's personality. The name, "Scout," came to Horovitz (Horovitz, 1999) for a variety of reasons, but mostly because the work with this client had been a constant challenge and adventure for Horovitz and for the client. Horovitz's methodology effected and transpired into informed decision making, improved communication and facilitated treatment objectives and goals. The work enabled other interdisciplinary team members to more aptly understand Scout and serve her needs since so many were puzzled by her behavior and communication style (or lack thereof).

Internet-Based Referrals

Finally, in the age of the World Wide Web (WWW), YouTube, Vonage, IChat, Skype, SightSpeed, and various other means of communication, it is wholly possible for art therapists to be contacted for their services. Again, it cannot be impressed enough that working (in person and in real time) is the most preferable and ethical form of treatment. However, this writer has been contacted for forensic interpretation via schools and law enforcement officials. Here, it is recommended that one tread lightly as analyzing data without the ability to directly observe a client is both dangerous and, in this author's opinion, suspect. If one has the ability to interact via the Internet with programs such as IChat or SightSpeed, then the client can be viewed in real time. However, the inability to pan in and actually see the details of the client working is not technically afforded at this juncture. In time, technology will improve and software programs will be developed so that an art therapist in, let's say, Rochester, New York will be able to communicate in real-time disaster situations (such as when workers cannot access areas – like the recent June, 2008 earthquake in Sangzao, China).

In October, 2007, a school psychologist and school principal contacted Horovitz. They had learned of her via the Internet and were perplexed by a recent drawing created by a 14 year-old male student. Given the propensity of Columbine disasters, and such disarming news, the administrators wanted to employ Horovitz's services to determine the welfare of this child. Because of their heightened concern, Horovitz agreed to view the artwork and offer them a consultation based on the information (or in this case, lack thereof) that they could (ethically) communicate. The result of that referral is below and hopefully will serve as a barometer for future art therapists when faced with similar inquiries for service.

Art Therapy Abbreviated Assessment – Internet Referral

<u>Referral Source:</u> **A.O. NCSP, School Psychologist; Ripley, New York School System**

<u>Date:</u> **October 30, 2007**

<u>Client:</u> **14.0 year-old male in the 8th grade**

<u>Art Therapist:</u> **Dr. Ellen G. Horovitz, ATR-BC, LCAT**

<u>Licenses:</u> **NYS License # 05 000467; NPI #1770790131**

Background and Reason for Referral

Due to confidentiality, there was no direct referral for this abbreviated assessment. The information provided by school psychologist, A.O., came by way of an Internet query for an evaluation of an attached artwork. The only information provided was the following from A.O. via an email communication on October 30, 2007:

> The art instructor told the students to zoom in on an insect and take it out of context. A teacher who was a casual observer initially brought it (N.B.: the drawing) to my attention.

Clearly, both the superintendent and the school psychologist (A.O.) were alarmed enough to contact the art therapist by email. Alas, it is difficult to analyze one piece of artwork, especially out of the context of its creation, since nonverbal body language or verbal associates to the artwork produced cannot be assessed; nonetheless, the art therapist will do her best to analyze the piece provided below given the context of both the query and the referral.

Analysis of the Work Produced

Figure 12.5 is an image created by a 14.0 male student currently in the eighth grade in the Ripley, NY School System. The artwork produced was not a free association but was derived from an art teacher's directive to create an insect by "zooming in on it and taking it out of context." Thus, should the image not bear a resemblance to the insect that was being modeled (and that information was also not provided), contextually, this might make sense.

On closer examination of the remodeled insect, much information (while a blind reading) can be derived:

The first and most obvious feature of this insect is its containment in a triangular shape. If in fact the insect is the amoeba-shaped, reddish-orange

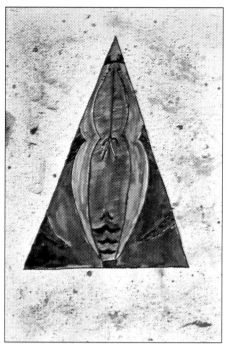

Figure 12.5. Student artwork of 14.0 male, eighth grade.

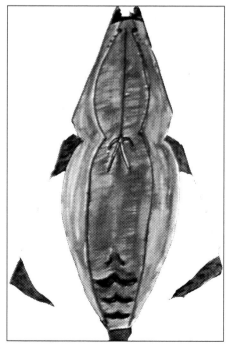

Figure 12.6. Insect out of its triangular habitat.

shape in the above drawing as indicated, then taken out of its triangular containment it would appear such as modified in Figure 12.6.

If indeed all of the parts above are part of the "zoomed-in insect," then this young boy attempted to contain all of its more aggressive parts. For example, when looking at an insect from the science Internet source below (Figure 12.7), the most aggressive parts of the insect featured are the mouthparts or abdominal areas (cercus) that are used as stout pincers or forceps. These areas are the passageways for the insect's meal and/or survival amongst other species.

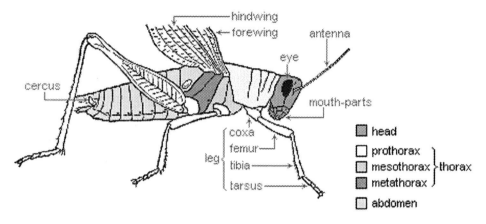

Figure 12.7. Source: http://www.kendall-bioresearch.co.uk/morph.htm

Given the fact that this insect's aggressive features are indeed contained, it points to one salient point: this young boy is attempting to harness any aggressive impulses that he may harbor if indeed the insect is to be viewed as any kind of self-portrait. (But given that this was an assignment, one can only hypothesize that he identified with this specific insect.) Indeed, the insect might also be viewed as his inability to survive his present environment since its survival is compromised by its containment.

Concluding Remarks

When viewed from an analytical standpoint in its triangular cocoon, the insect appears to be just below the surface; and in that, it may suggest that feelings are brewing that have not yet surfaced. The surrounding area around the triangular-contained insect appears to be a mottled, bloody-red splattered. While this might have been created due to experimental design, it is the only portion of Figure 12.5 that appears "out of control." The triangulated container for the insect smacks of controlled behavior on this young boy's part and suggests a heightened capacity for sublimation when working with art materials.

According to Cohen and Phelps (1985), Hammer (1980), Horovitz (1999, 2005, 2007), and Oster and Crone (2004), wedge shapes (such as triangles) have been seen in the victims of sexual abuse. Should this child have been victim to a sexually abusive relationship, it might explain the wedge-shaped container for his insect. With no evidence to support that hypothesis (in other theoretical constructs it would just be a container for the insect), according to the aforementioned sources, it might reflect this young man's desire for a nurturing, stable environment.

Developmentally, this adolescent young boy appears to be in the Pseudo-Naturalistic Stage of Development, approximately age 12–14 years, according to Lowenfeld and Brittain (1985). He is definitely functioning age appropriate and this artwork does not indicate any cognitive delays, neurological deficits, or pathological organicity.

Should this young man respond creatively and with concentration to art materials, and be in need of counseling, it is highly recommended that he be seen for an individual art therapy assessment to determine whether or not individual, group, and/or family art therapy is warranted.

_____   _____

Dr. Ellen G. Horovitz, ATR-BC, LCAT   Date

Conclusions Regarding Assessment, Diagnosis and Treatment, and Progress Notes

It is hoped that the above samples, as well as all the assessments in this book, will provide art therapists with the armament needed to make informed treatment decisions and be a respected member of an interdisciplinary team. While art therapy is a complementary and alternative form of treatment, it is also a science. Given that the field aspires to be taken seriously in the scientific community, it is our duty to respond in kind by communicating our findings in measurable terms (when possible) and to offer information that can be transliterated to an entire treatment team. If one demands to walk alongside other clinicians, it is imperative that one be able to speak the same language, formulate measurable clinical objectives, modalities, and goals that will dovetail with rest of the interdisciplinary team. Bearing that in mind, one also needs to know how to write a progress note, as well as an objective and modality.

Progress Notes — Procedures

A typical progress note, entered by a member of any discipline, should tell the problem or symptom being addressed, the precise treatment administered, the patient's reaction, and the patient's status at the time treatment was discontinued. All this need not entail a great deal of writing. It can be accomplished by carefully filling out flow sheets, graphs, etc. If the person making the progress note is a decision maker with authority to initiate or change treatment on his or her own professional judgment, the note should reflect the problem addressed and describe the reasons for undertaking, modifying, or discontinuing a particular treatment. (*The Record That Defends Itself*, Care Communications, Inc.)

Keep in Mind ➔ Progress Notes Should:

❏ Be keyed to goals and objectives: Be kept relevant to why patient is here receiving services.
❏ Show efforts of staff members: How does staff influence client? What treatment is going on and why?
❏ Indicate the course of treatment: Progress recording not process recording. Don't burden record with excessive verbiage.
❏ Show response to all treatment rendered: What works? What doesn't?
❏ Allow for midstream changes in treatment plans.

Following is an example of *objectives* and a sample report with *progress note* and *recommendations* for Matthew, a child with whom Horovitz worked for well over 4 years. (For more extensive understanding of this case, Horovitz created a movie of her work with this child that won the 2002 American Art Therapy Association James Consoli Video/Film Award for excellence in video production and contribution to the field).

Art Therapy Report/Objectives for 2004

Name: Matthew

Address:

Telephone:

DOB:

Date:

Period Covered: 2/3/04-4/27/04

At the end of last semester, Matthew had the following objectives in Art Therapy:

Matthew's Objectives

1. Continue to engage in conjoint weekly, hourly art therapy/speech therapy sessions in order to enhance Matthew's information processing while simultaneously increasing self-esteem and ego maturation.
2. Utilize storytelling materials for engaging in both co-creative play and simultaneous information processing. Since Matthew responds well to puppetry, continue utilizing this approach so that Matthew can find his own voice by May of 2004.
3. Proceed at a rate that matches Matthew's emotive level in order to enhance individuation, maturation, and cognitive functioning 50 percent of the time.

Matthew's Progress Note

Matthew continues to make use of merging his Art Therapy and Speech/Language Therapy in order to work on such issues as narrative production with a sequential framework, pragmatics, understanding comparative language in math word problems, and sentence repair. As well, he continues to work on metaphors, similes, and like topics as he engages in the Speech/Language Therapy. Kim Klotzbach, his speech/language therapist has done a remarkable job of fluidly integrating the speech/language projects into a creative and therapeutic format so that Matthew has been able to engage more readily towards his stated goals and objectives in both Art Therapy and Speech/Language Therapy.

Indeed, while the bulk of this semester's work has included the aforementioned topics, Matthew has simultaneously engaged in creative art projects both in and out of session. Below are some examples of this artwork. For example, using duct tape, Matthew created a thinking cap in order to aid him in his work with Ms. Klotzbach.

As well, Matthew created several other items, which aided him in working on narrative storytelling. While some of the storytelling work was written in session, the creative art projects were concertized while at home. This created continuity between sessions and aided Matthew in focusing and staying on task during his sessions with Ms. Klotzbach and Dr. Horovitz.

In his most recent session while playing a word game with Ms. Klotzbach that aided in math-related problems, Matthew created a puppet head from a balloon and masking tape. This project seemed to enliven Matthew and helped connect him in his work with the speech/language therapist.

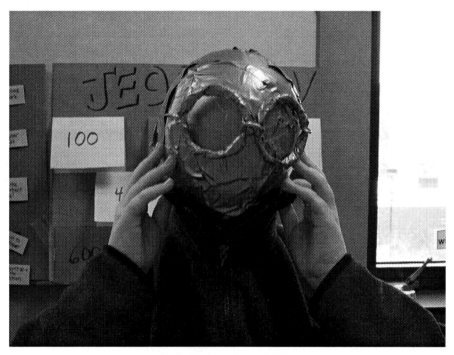

Figure 12.8. Matthew's "Thinking Cap."

Currently, Matthew is finishing a narrative story that he is illustrating outside of the therapy session. Below is a scene from the new story:

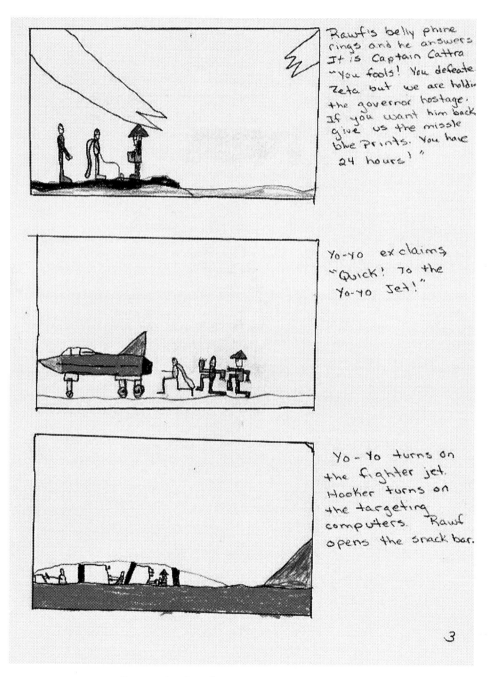

Figure 12.9. Matthew's Narrative Story Scene.

Recommendations

Matthew successfully integrates his artistic ability with his speech/language therapy and appears to be able to engage whether or not the art therapy is available to him. As a result, it appears as if Matthew has made significant gains in his work integrating the two disciplines. Therefore, it is recommended that Art Therapy be terminated at the end of this semester since Matthew seems capable of integrating his artistic abilities both in and out of the speech/language therapy. Because Matthew has worked with Dr. Horovitz for four years in this interdisciplinary approach, it is recommended that the termination of art therapy services be discussed with him to determine if he is comfortable with this proposal. Should this not be acceptable, then both his speech/language therapy supervisor and Dr. Horovitz will look at gradually reducing art therapy services. Matthew should be commended on his ability to integrate these combined services and integrate this information in such a creative manner.

_____   _____

Dr. Ellen G. Horovitz, ATR-BC, LCAT   Date

Process Notes – Procedures

A process note is an extensive note, comparable to a daily journal, which students keep on each patient serviced. Normally, those process notes are handed in to a site and/or academic supervisor on a weekly basis. In some clinical settings, the writings are reviewed and the supervisor makes comments to the supervisee directly on the written process note. This exchange is done *prior* to a supervisory meeting. The reason for this is so that the supervisor might extract pertinent information prior to the meeting to discuss within the confines of either individual or group supervision. It is to the student's benefit to be responsible for this exchange/dialogue on a continuing basis. Supervisors should not have to hound students for their journal/process note entries. In some settings, these notes are *expected* on a weekly basis. All of this depends on the placement and the administrative procedures.

Process notes need not be lengthy. Exceptionally pertinent material can generally be condensed and summarized with a one and a half to a two-page format. Moreover, sample drawings attached to the process note often clarifies the reading and offers increased insight to the eyes of the supervisor. So, by all means, feel free to include thumbnail sketches of the artwork that transpired.

In conclusion, it is hoped that this sashay into assessment, diagnosis, and treatment will serve the reader as an informed operating system and offer numerous templates from which the art therapist can operate within the various systems (e.g., educational, medical, research).

Remember, informed treatment rests on the enlightened percept of the examiner. It is hoped that these pages offer the reader a point of departure from which he or she can make educated decisions, ethical judgment, and salubrious treatment plans. In that, the authors wish you and your clients' good health.

APPENDICES

Appendix A

GENOGRAMS, TIMELINES, BEHAVIORAL OBSERVATIONS, AND PSYCHOSOCIAL INDICATORS

Client: Holly

DOB: 1978

CA: 27

Testing Dates: April 2, 2006

Administrant: Jane C. Adams

Assessments Administered: ATDA, HTP, PPAT

See Chapters 2, 7, and 9 respectively, for further examples regarding Holly

Behavioral Observations

Holly presented as a relaxed, outgoing individual who appeared quite comfortable with the process of completing the assessments. She demonstrated confidence during the drawing and discussion. She was cooperative and followed the directive with ease, making eye contact and conversing with the art therapist. Holly appears well-groomed, but she is also an extravagant dresser. She assisted in the clean-up process.

Genogram

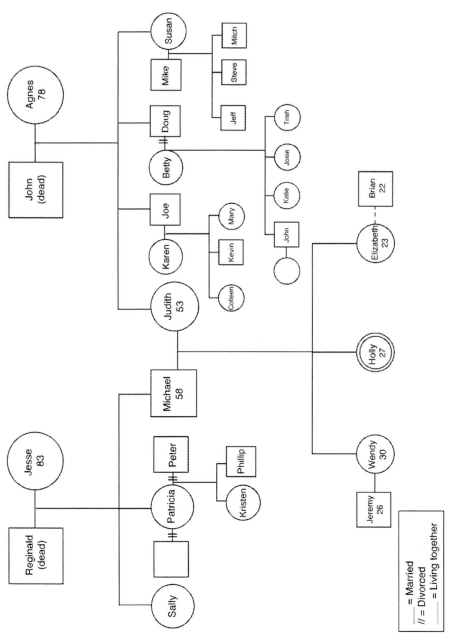

Figure A.1. Holly's Genogram.

Client: S

DOB: 2000

CA: 6 years old

Testing Dates: February 26, 2006; March 6, 2006; March 27, 2006

Administrant: Jacob Atkinson

Tests Administered: CATA, PPAT, SDT

See Chapters 1, 5, 9, and 10 for further examples regarding S.

Behavioral Observations

 S presents herself as an intelligent, well-groomed six year old, whose physical size is closer to that of a four-year-old. S's size is a result of her medically restricted diet of fruits and vegetables due to Eosinophilic Gastroenteritis. S's mother is Deaf and her father is hard-of-hearing, requiring S to learn and communicate by using both speech and sign language. S is friendly upon entering the clinic and even more so after her mother leaves.

History and Genogram

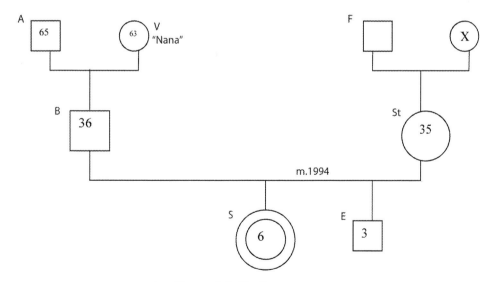

Figure A.2. S's Genogram.

Timeline

- 1-year-old and becomes ill
- 3-year-old S is diagnosed with Eosinophilic Gastroenteritis (EG) which currently only allows her to eat selected fruits and vegetables
- Her disorder has caused her many surgeries and tests
- 6-year-old S becomes frustrated with food restrictions
- S spent over a month at the KKI hospital in Baltimore for EG in November, 2005
- Returning to Hospital for a weekend checkup in April, 2006
- Mother is Deaf
- Father is hard of hearing
- Both paternal grandparents are Deaf

Identified Patient: M.S.

DOB: January 22, 1955

CA: 52

Administrant: Jaime Balduf

Testing Dates: January-April 2007

Assessments Administered: Bender Gestalt II

See Chapter 4 for a further example regarding S.

History and Genogram

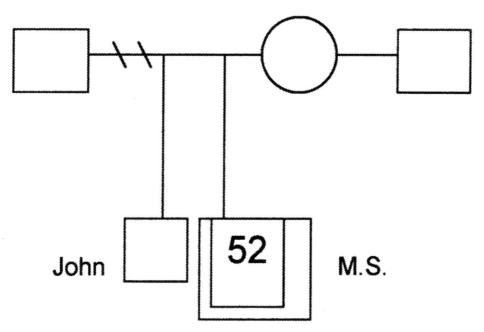

Figure A.3. M.S.'s Genogram.

Timeline

1955 – born into family with older brother

1970 – diagnosed borderline schizophrenic (symptoms more like ADD)

1977 – achieves GED

1978 – father dies, M.S. stops medication-no further signs of mental illness

1981–83 – attends technical school, degree in welding and auto mechanics

1983 – mother remarries

2000 – involved in MVA resulting in brain injury (subdural hematoma and coma for 1 month), receives extensive therapy, placed into mother's care

2001 – eye surgery

2000–05 – spends winters with family in Florida

2006–07 – first winter without family; stays in Rochester, NY

Behavioral Observations and Psychosocial Indicators

M.S. presented as a slightly disheveled, yet mild mannered and cooperative 52-year-old white male. His speech was blunt, fast, and at times, incoherent. This worker had to remind M.S. frequently to speak slowly and to repeat key words in order to improve communication and understanding. Once engaged, M.S. was quite talkative, especially when asked about his past. However, he would often become agitated and avoidant when his injury and emotional issues were discussed.

Individual art therapy sessions with M.S. took place within the art room of the Hickok Center for Brain Injury. He has been a member there for a few years as part of his service plan. M.S. became greatly invested in the art-making process and was very attentive to the directives this worker asked of him.

According to his files, M.S. was involved in a motor vehicle accident, resulting in a subdural hematoma and coma lasting for one month. He then received extensive cognitive and physical therapies and was put into his mother's care. His mother and stepfather have since remained as his primary support system. This winter has been the first for M.S. in which he did not join his parents on their vacation in Florida. M.S. currently takes medication for anxiety and acid reflux. He becomes anxious when his schedule is disrupted and fears being left alone. M.S. has had few friendships and appears introverted. His long-term memory is fairly in tact while his short-term memory is very poor. In reference to his injury, M.S. has no memory of his injury.

Client: Diane

DOB: June 5, 1962

CA: 44

Testing Date: October 14, 2006; October 18, 2006

Administrant: Day Butcher

Tests Administered: HTP

See Chapter 7 for a further example regarding Diane.

Behavioral Observations

Diane is white, non-Hispanic 44-year-old female of average height and build, well groomed and dressed. She was self-conscious about not being able to draw, but upon reassurance from the administrant, she proceeded with the first sequence of drawings. She did however draw each item (House, Tree, Person) very quickly with little thought or concentration on the image, with the exception of the two achromatic and chromatic person drawings. She talked freely about her husband and daughter and upcoming events in the neighborhood. She was very energetic and looked forward to the next two assessments.

Genogram

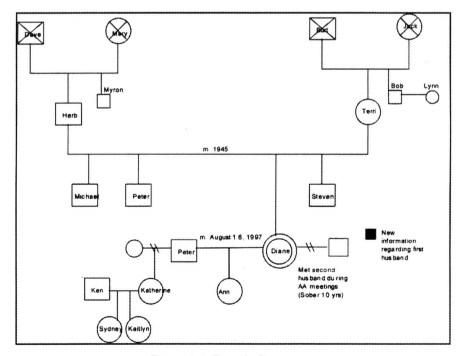

Figure A.4. Diane's Genogram.

Client: B

CA: 23

DOB: July 16, 1983

Testing Date: October 13, 2006; October 14, 2006; November 21, 2006

Administrant: Jenn DeRoller

Test Administered: Bender-Gestalt II

See Chapter 4 for a further example regarding B.

Behavioral Observations and Impressions

B was observed to be a very outgoing and happy person with a willingness and excitement to try new endeavors. Physically, she portrayed herself as overly worked and tired (as she called to reschedule our meeting for an hour later to take a nap). She entered the room, stating she was still exhausted but her overall appearance portrayed an awareness and energetic behavior. She was excited to begin the testing and eager to use the materials.

Although, initially she stated being tired, she came across as energetic and eager. She was inquiring and uncertain at first, remarking on the tests being administered and questioning the reasons for the tests. Overall, she was very concerned at the appearance of the pictures and whether she had done them "correctly," even though the administrant explained the pictures would not be judged by quality or quantity of the image. In the beginning of the test, B was very quiet while drawing her first image. She seemed overly focused on her drawing, but by the second drawing she appeared to relax and seemed comfortable in sharing past experiences and personal stories.

History and Genogram

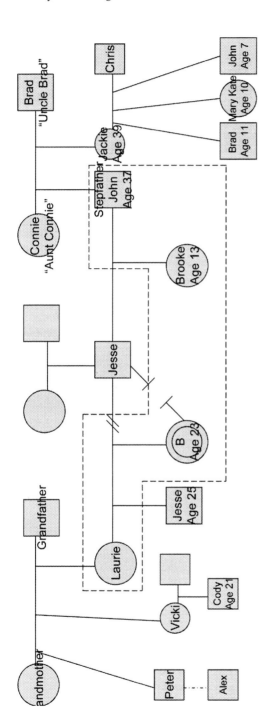
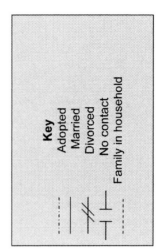

Figure A.5. B's Genogram.

Timeline

- Father was an alcoholic

- Parents divorced at 18 months old

- Mother remarried at age 9

- No contact with father

- Does not know family on father's side

- Stepfather and biological mother 9 years apart

- Age 13 – mother was hit by tractor trailer and was hospitalized for 3 months with an additional inpatient therapy for 3 months (two oldest Jesse and B left to take care of themselves)

- Age 18 – engagement to ES

- Age 18 – diagnosed with depression and anxiety (usually under control when medication taken and not under influence of alcohol)

- Age 20 – ended the engagement

- Age 22 – moved back home after graduation

Client: Nathan

CA: 26.9

DOB: April 5, 1979

Testing Date: April 2, 2006

Administrant: Sarah L. Eksten

Tests Administered: ATDA, KFD, SDT

See Chapters 1, 2, 8 and 10 for further examples regarding Nathan.

Psychosocial Indicators

Nathan is a 26-year-old Caucasian male who resides in a four-bedroom house with three other male roommates in Rochester, NY. He is in a long-term, committed relationship with his girlfriend, Jennifer, of 1.3 years. Nathan is currently pursing his doctoral degree in Microsystems at Rochester Institute of Technology (RIT). In addition to attending school, he works at RIT as a research assistant. Nathan was the first-born to Charlie and Jane in Baltimore, Maryland. His sister, Allison, was born two years later (see Genogram). Nathan moved to Rochester when he was 18 to attend RIT for his undergraduate degree in Microelectronic Engineering. Since then, he has resided in Rochester, except for one year when he worked in Belgium as a researcher.

Behavioral Observations

Nathan agreed to meet with the administrant. He presented himself as a well-groomed, attractive, cooperative individual, eager to complete the testing. He sat at the table patiently, pencil in hand, waiting for the instructions. Throughout the session, he gave meticulous attention to each art piece; although, it did not take him more than 15 minutes to complete any of the pictures. Before he announced he was complete with each picture, he would stop drawing, sit back in his chair, and look at his creation to make sure it was either complete, needed additions, or was to his liking. He would then look at the art therapist, turn the paper so that she could look at it from the correct angle, and wait patiently for questions. Nathan seemed a little tense when answering questions provided by the administrant, possibly because he wanted to make sure he provided the information she was looking for.

Timeline

1979 – Nathan is born

1981 – Allison is born

1997 – Nathan attends RIT for undergraduate school

2002 – Nathan begins Ph.D. program

2003 – Nathan moves to Belgium for one year

2004 – Nathan returns from Belgium; starts dating Jennifer; starts back at RIT for Ph.D. program

Genogram

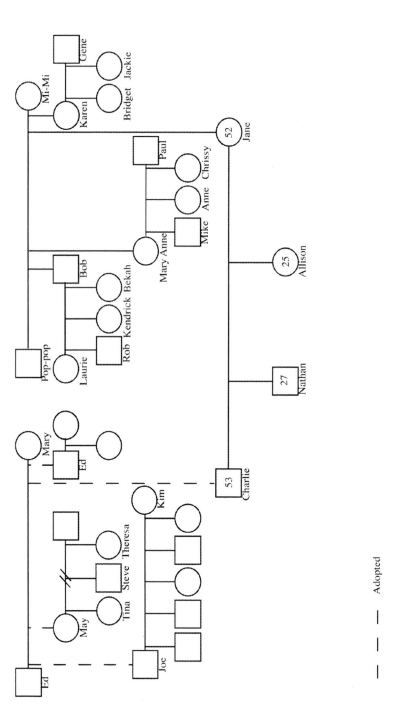

Adopted

Figure A.6. Nathan's Genogram.

Name: Adam

CA: 24.8

DOB: March 13, 1986

Administrant: Jordan M. Kroll

Test Date: November 19, 2006

Assessment: KFD

See Chapter 8 for a further example regarding Adam.

Psychosocial Indicators

Adam, a 24-year-old male, has known success throughout his life in virtually all of his undertakings. The youngest of three boys, he enjoyed popularity among both sexes growing up in Wisconsin. He currently works as a credit union representative in Michigan, and has past experience at a National Park and in the restaurant industry, including a management position. Not long before taking part in the Kinetic Family Drawing (KFD), he had recently split up with his girlfriend of over a year, though they remain friends. Adam feels he is in an "in-between" stage of his life, not knowing what the future holds. He came across as the type of person who either does his best at something, or else does not care to take it seriously. His preconception that he couldn't draw people, and especially not "people doing something," without using pictures, led to this KFD falling into the latter category. He stated upon completion that he "would rather have it look super real or really plain and playful." Here was an intelligent (college honors graduate) and creative (has published art and recorded music) individual who was intimidated at the prospect of producing a simple family drawing!

Genogram

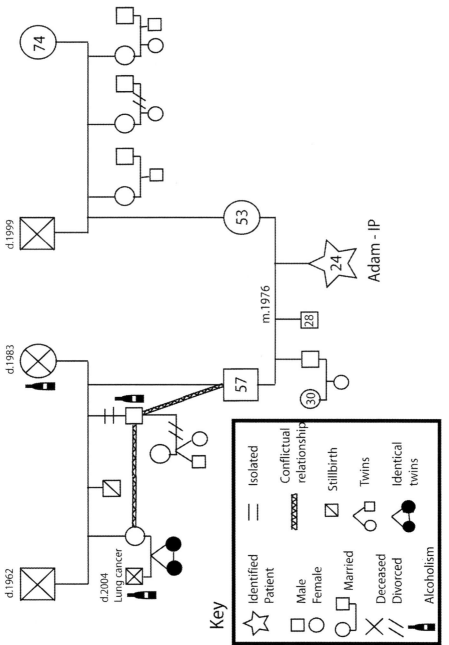

Figure A.7. Adam's Genogram.

Client: Lucy

DOB: August 25, 1978

CA: 28.2

Test Date: October 30, 2006

Administrant: Jordan M. Kroll

Tests Administered: CATA

See Chapter 5 for a further example regarding Lucy.

Psychosocial Indicators

Lucy presents an interesting case of personality as revealed through the art-making process. Born and raised in Montana, Lucy attended college in Seattle from 1997 to 2001. Following graduation, she moved to New York to pursue further education in the field of social work. She earned her Masters in 2003, and has been working full-time since then. During her schooling, Lucy remembers being interested in art, yet recalled receiving several "B"s in art classes and stated, "I don't get many 'B's."

Lucy's parents were divorced in 1986 and her mother moved to California, where Lucy spent her summers. During high school, she attended a Children of Divorce counseling class, which she said helped her work through her experience, and is currently of the opinion that everyone can benefit from some form of (preferably Christian) counseling. Of interest is the fact that her father and stepmother are both counselors. Lucy seemed to have positive, though somewhat distant relationships with her parents and siblings – one brother, one sister, and one stepsister. She last saw her mother, a self-proclaimed alcoholic, in the spring of 2006. Lucy is known presently to be a successful professional and a leader among a large circle of friends.

The evening of October 30, Lucy came straight from work to the test site. Though she hadn't eaten dinner, she said she was not yet hungry and her affect was charming, even energetic, as she smiled and popped bubbles with her gum.

Genogram

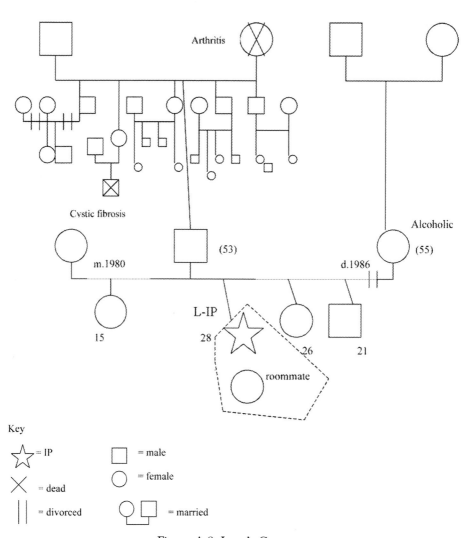

Figure A.8. Lucy's Genogram.

Client: L

DOB: January 20, 1958

CA: 49

Testing Date: April 1, 2007

Administrant: Barbara Murak

Tests Administered: ATDA, BATA, PPAT

See Chapters 2, 3, and 9 respectively, for further examples regarding L.

Behavioral Observations

The client is a petite, physically fit, single, 49-year-old woman. She was cheerful and cooperative during the testing process. Initially, the client was anxious about drawing skills, but by session's end the client communicated readily with the administrant, and trust was established. The art therapist noted that the client interrupted assessments many times with stories of her dating and sexual encounters.

History and Genogram

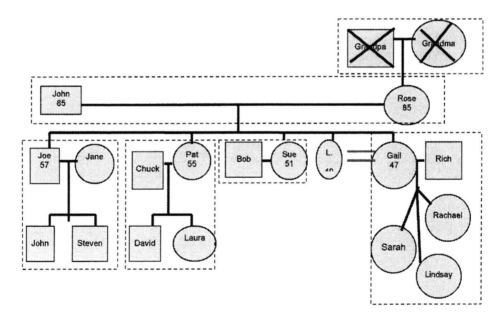

Figure A.9. L's Genogram.

Psychosocial Indicators

- Client: 49-year-old female, single and never married.

- During ages 18–28 yrs.: moved in and out of parents' house several times.

- Currently living in her deceased grandparents' house since 1986.

- Employment: works for brother, Joe, on family's rural farm. Volunteers at Ronald McDonald House in the city to enable socializing efforts.

- The client admits a conflicted relationship with her family, but remains close to younger sister, Gail.

- The client disclosed she frequently dates and has sex with men she meets through an Internet dating service.

- The client previously treated four times for depression/anxiety; last episode treated for 3 years and Zoloft. Currently no therapy or medication for one year.

- Maternal Grandmother put into psychiatric hospital for "nervous breakdown" and given electroshock (ECT) treatments.

- Client's sister has been on Celexa for several years; treated by family doctor; no psychotherapy.

- Belief system: the client was raised Catholic; now "spiritual, but not religious."

Client: Pam

DOB: August, 1954

CA: 52

Testing Dates: September 27, 2006; March 21, 2007; March 28, 2007

Administrant: Julie Riley

Tests Administered: BATA, FSA, SDT

See Chapters 1, 3, 6, and 10 for further examples regarding Pam.

Psychosocial Indicators

Pam is a single, white, 52-year-old female. Currently she lives with 5 housemates who help compose Pam's support system: these also include friends at DayHab, PRALID staff, and her advocate (literacy volunteer). Her remaining family, consisting of two older sisters, lives in New York State although not in the Rochester vicinity. Pam suffered a traumatic brain injury (TBI) following a head-on collision – motor vehicle accident (MVA) at the age of 16. Her boyfriend, the driver, died. Pam was in a coma for four months and received intensive medical attention and interventions. Between the time of the accident and 1986, her history is vague; but beginning in 1986 Pam rotated through several group homes in Connecticut until 1997 when she was moved to Rochester, NY, as advocated by her social worker. In 2002, she was monitored for a possible breast tumor. Also in September of 2002, Pam began stating intentions of self harm and suicidal ideations; though this was concluded to be attention-seeking behavior, she was recommended for counseling. During counseling, it was concluded that Pam was having difficulties around issues of mourning and loss of her life prior to accident, death of her boyfriend, and her deceased parents.

Behavioral Observations

Pam has a vibrant sense of humor and keen intellectual ability; she likes mathematics and occasionally speaks French (her mother was French). She is very fashion conscious and makes efforts to "look good." She uses a wheelchair due to left hemiparesis and subsequently has suffered visual impairment. Her memory is primarily limited to proximity and events prior to the MVA. Her medical chart indicates that she occasionally struggles with distinguishing reality from imagination; but in art therapy sessions this writer has been privy to imaginative expression on several occasions during which Pam was oriented in reality.

Timeline

8/54 – born

1969 – Parents Divorce

11/70 – MVA; head-on collision, severe head injuries, brain trauma right side (left hemiparesis), comatose for 4 months, Tracheotomy

Genogram

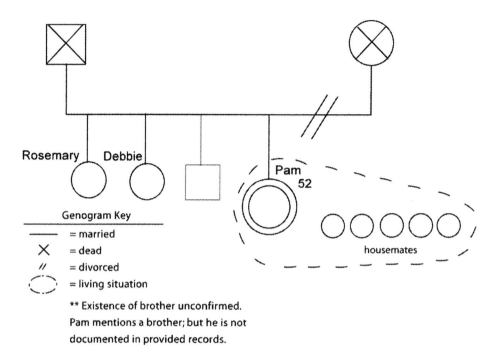

Figure A.10. Pam's Genogram.

Date unknown – Mother dies (heart attack)

4/86 – Admitted to Re-Entry Program at Golden Hill Health Care Center (Kingston, NY)

8/92 – Datahr ICF – Sweetcake Mountain group home (CT)

6/93 – Moved to Datahr ICF - Saw Mill group home (CT)

1/96 – Moved to Dorset Lane ICF group home (CT)

1997 – Moved to Rochester, NY

2002 – Monitored for possible breast tumor

9/2002 – Begins counseling due to statements of self harm and suicidal ideation

6/2006 – Referred to Nazareth Art Therapy Clinic

* It is unclear as to when Pam's father died; but at some point after mom dies and before being transferred to Rochester, NY, notations in paperwork indicate he is deceased.

Client: D

DOB: 05/27/86

CA: 22

Testing Dates: September 28, 2007

Administrant: M. Trinidad Selman P.

Tests Administered: CATA, KFD

See Chapters 5 and 8 respectively, for further examples regarding D.

Behavioral Observations

D is a third-year, undergraduate, international student at Nazareth College of the International Studies program. She came to the U.S. in year 2005 from Nepal, where all her family currently lives. She visited her family during the summer of 2007 and it was believed that she would not return to the States because she had a problem with her U.S. Visa. Nonetheless, the problem was solved and was able to come back. Yet, in the confusion, she lost the living space that she had originally shared with some friends. Thus, she is staying temporarily at a professor's house until spring semester of 2007. Throughout the assessment, she demonstrated very cooperative demeanor. However, she seemed to be very anxious due to the fact that she had to draw. Repeatedly, she commented that she didn't know how to do it, and that the last time she picked up an art material was in elementary school.

Genogram

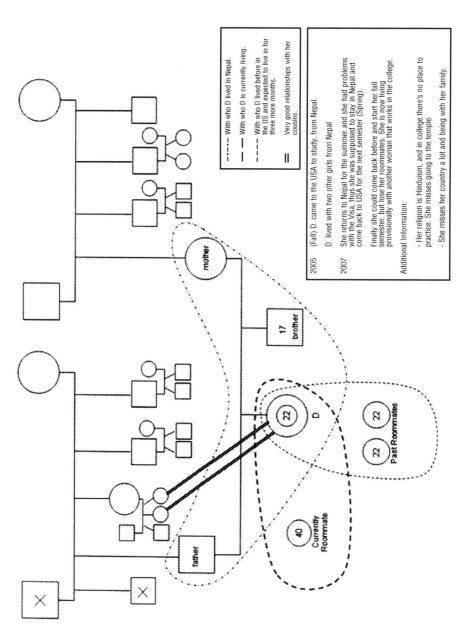

Figure A.11. D's Genogram.

Client: Karen

DOB: December 17, 1982

CA: 22

Testing Date: October 6, 2005

Administrant: Rachel N. Sikorski

Tests Administered: HTP

See Chapter 7 for a further example regarding Karen.

Psychosocial Indicators

Karen is a 22-year-old female who lives in her own apartment with a roommate and a small dog. She is an assistant manager of a retail store in the local mall, but is trying to decide what career path to choose. She studied both teaching and nursing during the four years she attended college. At 16, Karen graduated one year early from high school, and moved out of her mother and stepfather's home to live with her biological father. Prior to moving in with her father, Karen's relationship with his side of the family had been purely casual; she had seen him and his family on brief weekly visits since she was an infant.

Karen's birth was the result of an affair that her mother and father had while he was married to another woman. Her parents never married and she has two half-siblings close to her age from her father's first marriage, as well as two younger half-siblings from his current marriage (see history and genogram). Karen's mother married her stepfather, Aaron, when she was four. They subsequently had two children together. Aaron was an alcoholic and physically abused Karen's mother. Once, when she was five, her mother retaliated by stabbing him in the foot with a knife. This was followed by a one-night stay in a center for battered women and children. Shortly after, Karen and her mother moved back in with her maternal grandmother. Karen's mother went back to Aaron several weeks later, who had since quit drinking, and they bought their first home together.

Karen's mother had always been protective of her, especially because she struggled with asthma and therefore endured frequent hospitalizations as a child. Moreover, the two relied heavily on each other due to the mother's unstable relationships. They were often viewed as outcasts in the family, especially in the eyes of Karen's maternal grandfather, who Karen says "disowned" her and her mother. Her paternal grandparents also denied her status as a family member, and Karen did not have the opportunity to meet them until she moved in with her father at age 16.

After the birth of her younger sister, Kelly, Karen's relationship with her mother changed. She was no longer perceived as the "baby" of the family. Karen felt an undue amount of responsibility for the actions of her sister and misunderstood by her parents. She and her mother fought frequently (sometimes escalating to physical confrontation) until she moved out of the house. Karen believed that this change in environment was an improvement to their relationship.

Behavioral Observations

Karen presented as a friendly young woman, who made good eye contact. She was quiet, but not shy, and seemed comfortable talking to the writer about her history. In terms of physical appearance, Karen was short in stature, with shoulder-length blonde hair. She appeared well-groomed and was dressed neatly. Karen seemed to be unsure about her artistic skills; she communicated her discomfort both verbally and with the materials. Karen was quiet and seemed calm as she completed the response. She worked quickly, and depicted only minimal details in her work. Her timid nature and reserved expression may be a reflection of a lack of self-confidence or self-esteem.

History and Genogram

Infancy – Lives with single Mother and MGM; visits Father weekly
Close only to Mother/MGM side of family; MGF "disowns" her/her Mother

Age 4 – Mother marries Aaron

Age 5 – Witnesses physical abuse between parents; she and Mother endure a one-night stay in a center for battered women and children, then move in with MGM

Age 5 – After short separation from Aaron, move into new home together (alcohol use and PA stop)

Age 7 – Asthma under control; frequent hospitalizations stop

Age 8 – Birth of Kelly, frequent fighting with Mother begins; fighting turns physical as Karen gets older

Age 16 – Graduates one year early from high school, then moves in with Father

Age 16 – Meets PGP for first time, who had previously "disowned" her and denied her status as family

Age 21 – Gets her own apartment

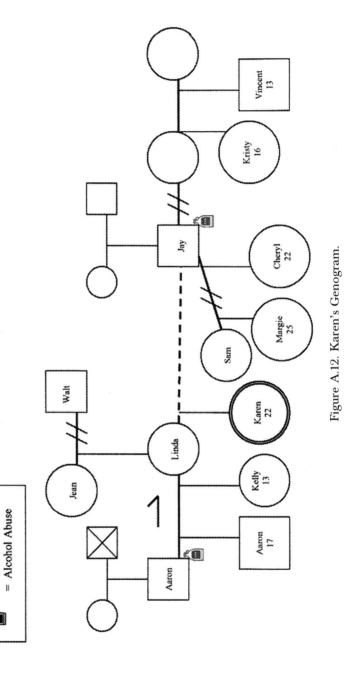

Figure A.12. Karen's Genogram.

Client: Sandy

DOB: May 23, 1972

CA: 33

Testing Date: April 9, 2006

Administrant: Rachel N. Sikorski

Tests Administered: CATA, FSA, PPAT

See Chapters 5, 6, and 9 respectively, for further examples regarding Sandy.

Psychosocial Indicators

Sandy is a 33-year-old female, who lives alone in her own home. She is a special education teacher at a school for multiply disabled young adults in wheelchairs. Sandy is the middle child in her family; her two younger brothers are Charlie and Paul, and her older brother and sister are William and Lisa. Sandy's sister, Lisa, recently divorced from her second husband and has moved back in with her parents along with her young daughter.

Growing up, Sandy's maternal grandmother lived with her family. She helped look after Sandy and her siblings while their parents tended to youngest brother, Charlie. He was very sick as a child, with a severe illness (undisclosed to this writer) that required frequent hospitalization. Sandy recalls how she and her siblings used to resent Charlie when they were children, because he was the main focus of their parents' attention at the time. Charlie recovered from his illness and Sandy's family began to spend more quality time together, especially during weekend trips to their private land in the country. When Sandy was nine years old, the family took a vacation to Disney World. This pleasant memory is significant for Sandy because it was the "one big trip" that she and her family shared together, outside of weekends spent on their land.

One event that had a tremendous impact on Sandy and her family was when younger brother, Paul, "came out" to the family about his homosexuality. She was 16 years old when her brother surprised her at work one day to give her a ride home. They drove around together for some time before Paul finally informed Sandy about his sexuality, which was a very difficult thing for her to accept. Sandy described her family at the time to have been "super-Catholic," and as such, the whole family had a hard time accepting Paul's news. Sandy's father was the only member of the family that supported Paul at the time and it would take years before the rest of the family would follow suit and accept Paul for who he was, regardless of his sexual orientation.

Behavioral Observations

Sandy presented as a friendly young woman, who made good eye contact. In terms of physical appearance, Sandy is tall and slim, with shoulder-length brown hair. She is well-groomed, has a natural look and wears little makeup. Sandy was open to making art and talking with the writer about her history; however, she limited the amount of detail that she shared about her family background. She seemed anxious and expressed some concern about performing well as an artist. Sandy's uncertainty about her artistic skills manifested itself several times throughout the session, most often in the form of frequent laughter and sarcastic comments that would address the quality of her artwork. Sandy completed each of the assessment tasks quickly and had a tendency to depict only minimal details in her work. Although she expressed enjoyment about making art and working with clay and paint during the assessment, Sandy spent very little time with these materials. Near the end of the session, she told the writer how uncomfortable she was with the lack of direction and structure for completing the art responses. Overall, it seemed that Sandy's reserved expressions, limited color selection and quick, simple responses to the art assessments may have been a reflection of her anxiety or a lack of self-confidence.

History and Genogram

Infancy – Paternal grandparents and maternal grandfather died before or during infancy; did not know them.

Childhood – Brother Charlie sick for most of his childhood; maternal grandmother lived with family and took care of the other children while parents tended to Charlie in the hospital.

Age 9 – Family vacation to Disney World, their "one big trip;" otherwise they spent weekends on private, family-owned land in the country for their "vacations."

Age 16 – Brother Paul "comes out" to family about his homosexuality; father was the only accepting one in their "super-Catholic" family. This "caused a rift" between Sandy and Paul for several years.

Age 23 – Maternal grandmother dies.

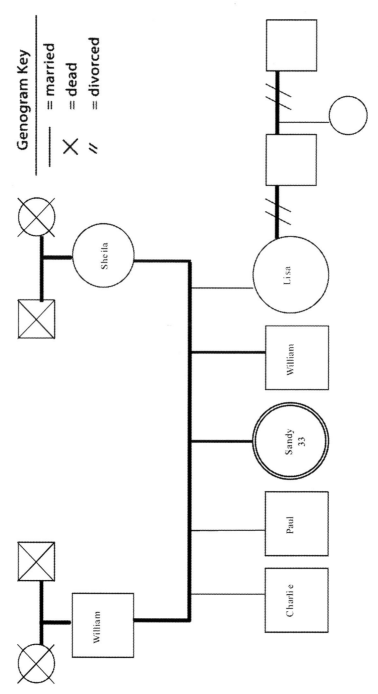

Figure A.13. Sandy's Genogram.

Client: Karla

DOB: September 11, 1985

CA: 22

Testing Date: September 24, 2007

Administrant: Luke M. Sworts

Tests Administered: BATA

See Chapter 3 for a further example regarding Karla.

Behavioral Observations

Karla appeared as an engaging and cheerful individual. Physically, she was attractive and well-groomed. Furthermore, she displayed a confidence in working with art materials and quickly selected the media of her choice. During the assessment Karla seemed apprehensive regarding the task, despite her known artistic skill. Karla's chosen medium, colored pencils, was age appropriate and offered her a precise tool for a certain degree of mastery (Oster & Crone, 2004). Though a trusting relationship was established, Karla had difficulty expressing herself comfortably and/or a large degree of confidence.

Psychosocial Indicators

A 22-year-old graduate student and full-time employee at Lowe's Hardware Stores, Karla identified herself as a Catholic. On the ensuing questions however, Karla indicated no change in her religious affiliation, no involvement with her church, and no religious practices of particular meaningfulness. This information suggests that Karla is a nonpracticing Catholic. Karla defined her relationship with God as a professional relationship, and then stated, "I don't know . . . I don't think I have one . . . it's just there." Karla added that she has not thought about God in a long time.

Karla suggested that the support of friends and family provides her with strength and meaning. Moreover, the idea of self-confidence and knowing that "everything will work out in the end . . . for a reason" was reassuring. In fact, Karla did not believe that God was involved in her problems or that she had ever felt a feeling of forgiveness from God. Lastly, Karla volunteered that she "only think[s] of God in birth and death situations."

History and Genogram

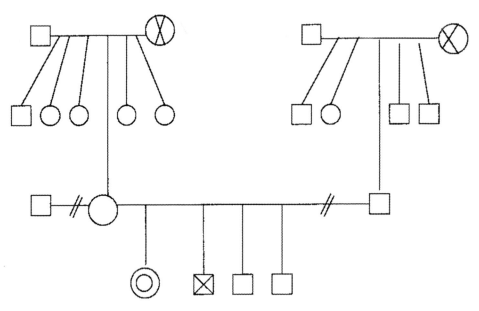

Figure A.14. Karla's Genogram.

Timeline

Age 3 – Birth and death of brother

Age 19 – Parents Divorce

Age 20 – Break-up with serious boyfriend

Age 21 – Graduate from college, start Graduate School

Client: Elizabeth

DOB: 1977

CA: 30

Testing Date: November 16, 2007

Administrant: Rebecca Ward

Tests Administered: KFD

See Chapter 8 for a further example regarding Elizabeth.

Psychosocial Indicators

Elizabeth is a white female, 30 years of age, who works full-time at a corporate job in international business. She has her own apartment and her extended family live in the same city. She is the oldest of five children, three of them are half siblings. At the age of four, Elizabeth's abusive father abandoned the family and her mother remarried two years later. Elizabeth avoided further questions about the type of abuse she had been subjected to. Elizabeth's stepfather adopted Elizabeth and her sister; her parents went on to have three more children.

Elizabeth currently has a very close relationship with her sister, Laurelle, and with her father. Elizabeth and her mother have not been as close the past ten years and this relationship is the cause of much anxiety in her life. Although Elizabeth and her extended family all live in the same city, she doesn't visit or communicate with her parents very often.

Behavioral Observations

Elizabeth presented as a friendly, well-dressed woman who appears younger than her actual age. She was very compliant to the directive and only made a few joking comments about her drawing abilities.

Genogram

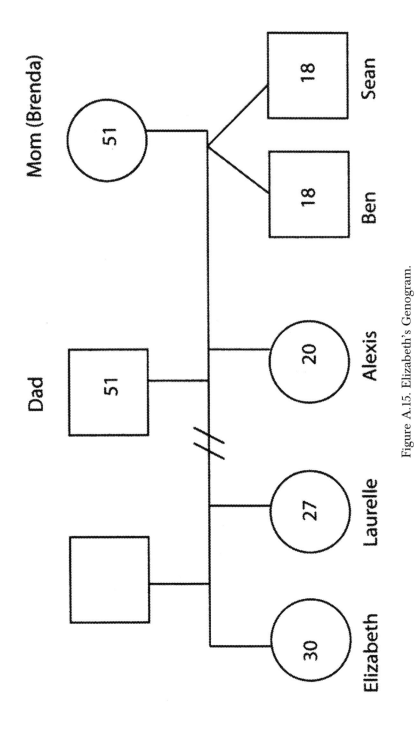

Figure A.15. Elizabeth's Genogram.

Appendix B

OUTLINE FOR DEVELOPMENTAL STAGES IN ART BASED ON *CREATIVE AND MENTAL GROWTH*

Lowenfeld and Brittain

I. <u>Scribbling</u> – First Stages of Self Expression (2–4 years)
    (A child should never be diverted from scribbling)
    A. Types (Sequence)
        1. Disordered (about 2 years) – uncontrolled
        2. Controlled – longitudinal type (approx. 2 1/2 years) – control over emotions
        3. Controlled – geometric scribble, circular type – motions changed because of mastery of previous type
        4. Naming of scribbling – change from the kinesthetic approach (or one involving motions) to an imaginative one involving pictures
    B. Concepts of figures – none except kinesthetically
    C. Concepts of space – none
    D. Meaning of color – no conscious use; subordinate roll in scribbling
    E. Clay work
        1. Plasticene of figures (clay with oil base) used
        2. Beating and pounding of clay – corresponds to disordered period in scribbling
        3. First conscious approach of shaping the clay corresponds to the controlled state in scribbling
        4. Naming of lumps of clay – "This is a train," etc.
    F. Stimulation topics – none during the first stages of scribbling – almost any when approach to art projects is purely imaginative
    G. Media
        1. Large black crayons
        2. Smooth paper
        3. Finger painting
        4. Colored crayons (four colors)
        5. Plasticene

II. <u>Preschematic Stage</u> – First Representational Attempts (ages 4 to 7)
    (A relationship with reality has been achieved; the child constantly searches for new concepts of man and his environment which will later result in established individual schema.)
    A. Child uses his active knowledge or what actively motivated him in his drawings
        1. Representative symbols formed
            Def. – A representative symbol consists of geometric lines, which when isolated from the whole, lose their meaning

B. Figure Concept
  1. Head feet representations
  2. Use of body – with or without arms
  3. Head, body, legs, and arms included – with or without characterizations
C. Space Concept – (Space is everything outside the body)
  1. Earliest organizations not subject to any law
  2. Relationships between objects expressed not evident
  3. No experience of Child's place in the environment
D. Significance of Color
  1. No relationship to reality
  2. Emotional appeal only
E. Clay work
  1. Pulling out from lump of clay – lesser consciousness of the form
  2. Adding to – more consciousness of forms
  3. No desire for decoration as long as child searches for a form concept
F. Stimulation Topics
  1. Activation of passive knowledge mainly to self
    a. Use of "I" and "My"
    b. Use of "What", "How", Where", and "When"
       Ex. I and my Mother (sizes)
           I am Brushing My Teeth (teeth)
           My Birthday Present (emotional relationship)
G. Media
  1. Crayons (eight colors)
  2. Clay (water base)
  3. Powder paint (or poster)
  4. Thick large bristle brushes
  5. Large sheets of absorbent paper
  6. Unprinted newsprint
  7. Finger painting (with reservations)
III. Schematic – Achievement of a form concept (7 to 9 years)
   (Discovery of definite concept of man and his environment; self assurance through repetition of form symbols: "schema." In pure schema no intentional experience is expressed, only the thing itself: "the man," "the tree," and so forth.)
A. Pure schematic representation is one with no intentional experience represented. The schema of an object is the concept at which the child has finally arrived, which represents the child's active knowledge of the object.
  1. Particular experience manifested through deviations in his schema
    a. Exaggeration and omission of important parts
    b. Neglect or omission of unimportant or suppressed parts
    c. Change of symbols of emotionally significant parts
  2. Origin of deviations lies in autoplastic experience (feelings of the bodily self, importance of value judgments with regard to certain parts, or in the emotional significance which this part has for the child)

B. Figure Concept
(Human schema – form concept of the figure at which the child has finally arrived, after long struggles of searching during the preschematic stage)
1. Deviations in schema occur, i.e., exaggeration, omission, change of symbols

C. Space Concept
1. Base-line – first definite space concept. Discovery of being a part of the environment: assumption for cooperation and correlation.
   a. Base-line expresses base and terrain
2. Subjective space representations – all representations in which an emotional experience forces the child to deviate from his space schema.
   a. Base-line continues to function
      Folding over – space schema created by drawing objects perpendicular to the base-line (usually used by egocentric children)
      Space and Time Representations – different time sequences in a single space
      X-ray pictures – inside and outside depicted simultaneously whenever the inside is emotionally more significant than the outside
      Mixture of plane and elevation – viewing some objects in picture plane a top and some from a side view
   b. Subjective spatial relationship – base-line dropped. Emotional experience is so strong that overpowers feeling of being part of the ground

D. Meaning of Color
Relationship between colors and objects established – objective relationship occurs. Color schema will not change unless in definite emotional experience induces the deviation in color.

E. Modeling – good at this level because of its plasticity; it lends itself for deviations in concepts better than other media
1. Analytic – pulling parts out from the whole
2. Synthetic – putting single representative together to from a whole

F. Design – (no conscious approach – no fundamentals taught). Innate sense of design seen in repetition of set schema.

G. Stimulation topics – must use we – some action – and where
Ex. We are skating on the pond (action)
    When we visit the hospital (x-ray)
    Eating breakfast (profile view)
    When we went to visit the market (space – time)

H. Media (techniques)
Important techniques should:
1. Be developed by the child
2. Should make their own contributions
3. Not be so numerous that they overpower the child
   a. Colored crayons
   b. Colored chalk
   c. Powder paint (tempera or poster)

      d.   Large paper (18x24)
      e.   Hair brushes (squirrel, camel, etc.)
      f.   Clay

IV. <u>The Dawning Realism</u> – <u>Gang Age</u> (9 to 12 years)
(The child's confidence in his own creative powers is for the time shaken by the fact that he is becoming conscious of the significance of his environment.)

  A. Characterized by removal from schema or generalizations
     1. Every part of a child's drawing now has meaning and retains it even when separated from the whole
     2. Group friendships or gangs of the same sex are common
     3. Lack of outside cooperation evident
     4. Discovery of social independence

  B. Figure concept
     1. Child concerned with representing characteristics of sex, i.e., girls with dresses, boys with trousers
     2. Greater interest in the "how" or details
     3. Increased stiffness in drawing – less feeling for action
     4. Through growing awareness of a visual concept the child no longer uses exaggeration, neglect, or omission as much as previously – but rather concentrates on details. As yet there is no interest or concept of folds or wrinkles in clothes – hemlines are still straight.

  C. Space concept
     1. Plane between the base line is discovered – space between base line is meaningful
     2. Sky is now drawn all the way to the ground
     3. Child becomes conscious of the overlapping of one object with another
     4. Group work of special significance
        Child should have the feeling that he could not have achieved singly what he can accomplish as a group

  D. Color subjective stage – color is used with regard to subjective experience. No longer is the color-object relationship used.
     1. There is the place in the elementary school classroom for the teaching of color wheels
     2. Emphasis on the emotional approach to color
        Ex. Dull colors used for the atmosphere of slums – bright colors for desirable housing conditions

  E. Modeling – modeled pieces are not intended for firing. A child's individual thinking should not be sacrificed to a mere technique.
     1. Self – expression is still the prime factor in modeling
     2. Introduction to pottery

  F. Design – First conscious approach to decoration now occurs. Crafts and design should be completely integrated.
     1. Design should grow out of the material
     2. Scientific or planned design should not be used here
     3. Crafts should never be separated from design

      4.   Realistic approaches to design should not be used

      5.   Experimentation encountered with new materials and techniques

G. Stimulation topics

      1.   Topics need to relate spatial experiences of the newly discovered plane to the self, i.e., Playing football

      2.   Topics need to inspire cooperation or the representation of scenes in which cooperation is important

         Subjective method – individual experiences of cooperation – decorating a Christmas tree

         Objective method – deals with group work – a whole group works on a project – We are all making a puppet show

      3.   Overlapping planes – (cut paper is an excellent medium)

         In the Train

      4.   Media – with the discovery of the plane the child now needs to use media to allow him to fill in spaces

         a.   Colored paper (paper cutting)

         b.   Poster paint – hair brush

         c.   No crayons (too linear)

         d.   Flat colored chalk

         e.   Clay

         f.   Finger paint

         g.   Paper mache

         h.   Linoleum, wood, metal

V. Pseudorealistic Stage – Stage of Reasoning (12–14 years)

(Characterized by a change in the imaginative activity of the child from that of the unconscious to one of critical awareness. This change accompanies physical changes in the body. There is also a shift of emphasis from the creating process to the product. Visual and nonvisual types appear – the former spectators in their environments and the latter always involved in the action. Love for action and dramatization is quite evident.)

A. Division of approaches into the visual and the nonvisual

B. Figure Concept

      1.   Introduction to joints – more desire to express action

      2.   The visually minded child notices folds in the garments, lights, and shadows on objects

      3.   Child wants to use correct proportion – exaggeration less frequently used

      4.   Nonvisual child concentrates on details in which he is emotionally interested. He will use exaggeration to express these parts.

C. Space concepts – Development of two concepts

      1.   Visual – optical changes in space

         Diminishing of distant objects

         Meaning of the horizon line

         Three-dimensional quality of space

      2.   Nonvisual – retrogression to the vase – line expressions

         Uses space only for the expression of self

D. Color – effect on two groups
    1.   Visuals – changes in color because of distance and mood
        Color in its changing effects
E. Modeling – Shift from modeling or the unconscious approach to three-dimensional expression to the conscious called sculpturing
    1.   Easier to arrive at in clay than in a painting technique
    2.   Visuals and nonvisuals face the same problem since environment is excluded
F. Design – The visually minded is concerned with the aesthetic function while the nonvisual is concerned with emotional abstractions
    1.   Conscious approach to stylizing of industrial products
    2.   Function of different materials and simple designs related to them
G. Stimulation topics
    1.   Posed models (clay)
           A Girl Reading
           Thinking at a Desk
    2.   Action (imagination)
           Fishing in a Pond
    3.   Proportion
           Climbing a Tree
    4.   Color
           Personification of Color
           Cold in Winter
    5.   Murals
           From – To as from Atlantic to Pacific Coast
           Frieze – Topics with continuity as Fruit Harvest
    6.   Design
           Characterize Profession by means of a symbolic design – shoemaker, tailor, etc.
           Abstract designs from different materials
H. Media (techniques)
   Water color (first introduced here – good for atmospheric changes)
   Poster paint
   Mixed techniques – watercolor and tempera
   Brushes – hair and bristle
   Linoleum
   Clay
   Wood, metal, stone, etc. (design materials)

SCRIBBLING STAGE – TWO TO FOUR YEARS

Characteristics	Human Figure	Space	Color	Design	Motivation Topics	Materials
1) Disordered. Kinesthetic experience. No control of motion.	None	None	No conscious approach. Use of color for mere enjoyment without any intentions.	None	Through encouragement. Do not interrupt or discourage or divert child from scribbling.	Large black crayon. Smooth paper. Poster paint. Finger paint only for maladjusted children. Clay.
2) Controlled. Repeated Motions, establishment of coordination between visual and motor activity. Control of motions. Self-assurance of control through deviations of type of motions.	None	None or only kinesthetically	Same as above.	None	Same as above.	Same as above.
3) Naming. Change from Kinesthetic to imaginative thinking. Mixing of motions with frequent interruption.	Only imaginatively by the act of naming	Purely imaginatively	Color used to distinguish different meanings of scribbling.	None	In the direction of the child's thinking by continuing the child's story.	Colored crayons. Poster paint. Clay. Felt-nibbed pen.

The Art Therapists' Primer

PRESCHEMATIC STAGE – FOUR TO SEVEN YEARS

Characteristics	Human Figure	Space	Color	Design	Motivation Topics	Materials
Discovery of relationship between drawing, thinking, and environment.	Circular motion for head, longitudinal for legs and arms. Head-feet representations develop to more complex form concept. Symbols depending on active knowledge during the act of drawing.	Self as center with no orderly arrangement of objects in space: "There is a table, there is a door, there is a chair." Also emotional relationships: "This is my doll."	No relationship to nature. Color according to emotional appeal.	No conscious approach.	Activating of passive knowledge related mainly to self (body parts).	Crayons, clay, tempera paints (thick), large bristle brushes, large sheets of paper (absorbent).

SCHEMATIC STAGE – SEVEN TO NINE YEARS

Characteristics	Human Figure	Space	Color	Design	Motivation Topics	Materials
Formulation of a definite concept of man and environment. Self assurance through repetition of form symbols, schemata. In pure schema no intentional experience is expressed, only the thing itself: "The man, the tree," etc. Experiences are expressed by deviations from schema. Use of geometric lines.	Definite concept of figure depending on active knowledge and personality, through repetition: figure schema. Deviations expressing experiences can be seen in – 1) Exaggeration 2) Neglect or omission of unimportant parts. 3) Change of symbols	First definite space concept: base line. Discovery of being a part of environment: important for cooperation and reading. Base line expresses – 1) Base 2) Terrain Deviations from base line express experiences. Subjective space: 1) Folding over (ego-centric) 2) Mixed forms of plan and elevation 3) X-ray pictures 4) Space-time representations	Discovery of relationship between color and object; through repetition color schema. Same color for same object. Deviation of color schema shows emotional experience.	No conscious design approach.	Best motivation concentrated on action, characterized by we, action, where. Topics referring to – 1) Time sequences (journeys, traveling stories) 2) X-ray pictures (inside and outside are emphasize), factory, school, home, etc.	Colored crayons. Colored chalk. Tempera, poster paint. Large paper. Bristle and hair brushes. Clay: 1) Synthetic 2) Analytic

STAGE OF DRAWING REALISM – NINE TO ELEVEN YEARS

Characteristics	Human Figure	Space	Color	Design	Motivation Topics	Materials
Gang age. Removal from geometric lines (schema). Lack of cooperation with adults. Greater awareness of the self and of sex differences.	Attention to clothes (dresses, uniforms) emphasizing difference between girls and boys. Greater stiffness as result of egocentric attitude and the emphasis on realistic lines. Removal from schema. Tendency toward details (clothes, hair, and so forth). Removal from schema.	Removal from base line expression. Overlapping. Sky comes down to base line. Discovery of plan. Filling in space between base lines. Difficulties in spatial correlations as result of egocentric attitude and lack of cooperation.	Removal from objective stage of color. Emphasis on emotional approach to color. Subjective stage of color. Color is used according to subjective experience.	First conscious approach toward decoration. Acquaintance with materials and their function.	Self-awareness stimulated by characterization of different dresses and suits (professions). Cooperation and overlapping through group work. Subjective cooperation through type of topic: "We are Building a House." Objective cooperation through team work.	Paper cutting. Crayons. Poster paint. Flat, colored. Chalk. Clay. Paper-mache. Wood. Collage materials. Metal. Prints.

PSEUDO-NATURALISTIC STAGE – ELEVEN TO THIRTEEN YEARS

Characteristics	Human Figure	Space	Color	Design	Motivation Topics	Materials
Developed intelligence, yet unawareness. Naturalistic approach (unconscious). Tendency toward visual- or nonvisual-mindedness. Love for dramatization and action.	Joints. Visual observation of body actions. Proportions. Emphasis on expression by nonvisually minded.	Urge for three-dimensional expression. Diminishing size of distant objects. Horizon line (visually minded). Environment only when significant (nonvisually minded).	Changes of color in nature for distance and mood (visually minded). Emotional reaction to color (nonvisually minded).	First conscious approach to stylizing. Symbols for professions. Function of different materials, with related designs.	Dramatic actions in environment. Actions from imagination and posing (with meaning, like scrubbing). Proportions through emphasis on content. Color moods.	Water color. Gouache (water color and tempera). Poster paint. Bristle brush. Hair brush. Clay. Linoleum. Paper-mache. Textiles. Wood.

CRISIS OF ADOLESCENCE – THIRTEEN TO SEVENTEEN YEARS

Characteristics	Human Figure	Space	Color	Design	Motivation Topics	Materials
Critical awareness toward environment. Three groups: 1) Visual Type: Intermediaries: eyes. Creative concern: environment, appearance. 2) Haptic Type: Intermediary: body. Creative concern: self-expression, emotional approach to subjective experiences. 3) In-betweens: Reactions are not definite in either direction. Creative concern: abstract.	Visual Type: Emphasis on appearance, proportion. Light and shadow. Depiction of momentary impressions. Naturalistic interpretations of objective validity. Haptic Type: Emphasis on inward expressions. Emotional qualities. Proportion of value. Individual interpretations. Depiction of character.	Visual Type: Perspective representations. Apparent diminution of distant objects. Atmosphere. Appearance. Mood. Three-dimensional qualities. Light and shadow. Horizon line. Haptic Type: Perspective of value with relation to the self. Value relationship of objects. Base-line expressions.	Visual Type: Appearance of color in nature. Color reflections. Changing qualities of color in environment, according to distance and mood. Analytic attitude. Impressionistic. Haptic Type: Expressive, subjective meaning of color. Local color when significant. Color changes with emotional and psychological significance.	Visual Type: Aesthetic interpretation of form, balance, and rhythm. Decorative quality of design. Emphasis on harmony. Haptic Type: Emotional design of abstract quality. Functional design. Industrial design.	Visual and haptical stimulations. Environment and figure. Appearance and content. Posing, with interpretations. Sketching. Sculpture. Graphics. Design. Painting. Mural.	Sketching in crayon, oil paint, tempera, conte, water color. Easel painting. Mural. Sculpture in clay, plaster, etc. Casting. Wood. Metal. Stone. Graphics.

ADOLESCENCE ART – THIRTEEN TO SEVENTEEN YEARS

Characteristics	Human Figure	Space	Color	Design	Motivation Topics	Materials
Ambition. Energy. Romantic ideals. Introspection. Peer-group pressures. Sexual awakening.	Action. Participation. Self-identification or empathy. Clothing. Costume. Dance and rhythm.	Visual perspective or perspective of value.	Sophisticated. Not necessarily naturalistic.	As integral part of function. In furniture, clothing, ornament, architecture, home style, site, landscaping, interior decoration. Appreciation. Abstract. Cartoons.	Self, home, community, nature, industry. Explore materials rather than emphasize technical excellence. Develop sensitivity. Excursions.	Any materials that contribute to further growth or adult use. All previous materials, plus photography, ceramics, wood (constructing and carving). Natural materials.

Eras/Ages	Erikson	Piaget	Kohlberg	Lowenfeld/ Brittain*	Horovitz
Infancy (0–1.5 yrs)	Basic Trust vs. Basic mistrust (hope)	Sensorimoter Stage		Scribble Stage: Beginning of Self-Expression (age 0-2 years)	
Early Childhood (2–6 yrs)	Autonomy vs. Shame & Doubt Initiative vs. Guilt (Purpose)	Preoperational or Intuitive	*Preconventional Level* 1. Heteronomous Morality	Preschematic Stage: First Representations (4–7 yrs)	
Childhood (7–12 yrs)	Industry vs. Inferiority	Concrete Operational	2. Instrumental exchange *Conventional level* 3. Mutual Interpersonal relationships	The Schematic Stage: Formed Concepts (age 7–9 yrs)	
Adolescence (13–21yrs)	Identity vs. Role Confusion (fidelity)	Formal Operational	4. Social System and Conscience	The Gang Age: Dawning Realism (age 9–12 yrs)	
Young Adulthood (21–35 yrs)	Intimacy vs. Isolation (Love)		*Postconventional Principled Level* 5. Social contract, individual rights	Pseudo-Naturalistic Stage: Age of Reasoning (age 12–14 yrs.)	
Adulthood (35–60 yrs)	Generativity vs. Stagnation (Care)			Adolescent Art: Period of Decision (14–17 yrs)	
Maturity (60 +)	Integrity Vs. Despair (Wisdom)		Universal Ethical Principles		Adult Stage: Formation in the World (age 18– adulthood

					Artistic Stage: Formed Art Any age (generally in adolescent through adulthood)

[1] Re: the Stages of Development as outlined by Lowenfeld and Brittain: please see below:

[1] While Lowenfeld and Brittain do not describe this as a stage, **Brain Injured Stage** can occur at any age, and I have described this stage in my lectures as consisting of organic qualities, where objects float on the page (e.g., lack of order and ungrounded quality to the artwork is pervasive in the representations, be they two or three-dimensional in design.)

As well, since they do not hallmark the **Adult or Artistic Stages of Development**, Horovitz does, since she feels that these stages vary dramatically from the Adolescent period, the last stage, which they described.

Appendix C

SAMPLE FORMAT

Art Therapy Diagnostic Assessment

Name:
Address:

DOB:
CA:
Testing Dates:
Tests Administered: Belief Art Therapy Assessment (BATA)
                     Kinetic Family Drawing (KFD)
                     Cognitive Art Therapy Assessment (CATA)
                     House-Tree-Person Test (HTP)
                     Silver Drawing Test of Cognitive and Creative Abilities (SDT)
                     Formal Elements Art Therapy Scale (FEATS)
                     Bender Visual Motor Gestalt Test
Administrant:

Behavioral Observations and Impressions:

Belief Art Therapy Assessment (BATA) Results:

Kinetic Family Drawing (KFD) Results:

House-Tree-Person Test (HTP) Results:

Cognitive Art Therapy Assessment (CATA) Results:

Silver Drawing Test of Cognitive and Creative Abilities (SDT) Results:

Formal Elements Art Therapy Scale (FEATS) Results:

Bender Visual Motor Gestalt Test Results:

Conclusion and Summation:

Administrant's Signature   Date

Appendix D

GUIDELINES FOR RECORDABLE, SIGNIFICANT EVENTS FOR ALL AGED CLIENTS IN CARE

NOTE: IF THERE IS EVER ANY DOUBT AS TO WHETHER AN EVENT SHOULD BE RECORDED OR HOW TO RECORD A SIGNIFICANT EVENT, CONTACT YOUR SUPERVISOR.

1. All incidents: restraints, accidents, AWOLs, drug reactions, missed medications, substance abuse, suicide attempts, assaults, fire setting, property damage, weapons possession, injury

2. Suicidal/self-destructive ideation/verbalization

3. Client removal (e.g., from milieu or classroom to crisis center)

4. Illness, complaints of illness, seizure, "normal" drug side effects (e.g., drowsiness), medical concerns

5. Client absconds

6. Interactions with significant others (e.g., phone call with parent)

7. Disclosure of significant feelings/insights

8. Treatment breakthroughs: major and minor

9. Strikingly uncharacteristic behavior

10. Client fights

11. Threats of destructive acts

12. Fantasies/Hallucinations

13. Sexual Interactions/Behavior/Acting out/Abuse/Concerns

Appendix E

MENTAL STATUS CHECKLIST

Chief Complaint: Name: Date:
                                         Medical Record No:
                                         Address:

Referred By: Phone:
Date of Birth:

Time Evaluation Began: Marital Status:
Gender:
Ended:

                                         Current Living Status
                                         [note if homeless]

                                         Legal Status on Arrival
                                         (if taken to Ed):

Primary Care Physician and Phone:

Data Required by the Office of Mental Health Primary Language: Race: Specific Cultural Identity: Current Disabilities:

ALERTS: Note risk factors identified (e.g., Danger to Self/Others, Escape Risk, Physical Health Needs/Conditions, Criminal Procedure Law Status, Previous known Adverse Reactions to Medications, etc.)

Insurance:
Presenting Problem/Illness/Family/Social and Psychiatric History
Include who called the team, what their concerns are, and what they want the team to do. Include a brief description of events leading to this presentation. Include current psychiatric symptoms and time frames in which client has experienced them, psycho-social stressors, medical problems, medications, substance abuse, sexual abuse, legal issues, employment, culture, psychiatric treatment, social supports, etc.

_____
_____
_____
_____
_____
_____
_____
_____
_____
_____

_____
_____
_____
_____
_____
_____
_____
_____
_____
_____
_____

Name:

Medical Record Number: Date:

_____
_____
_____
_____
_____
_____
_____
_____
_____
_____

Name:

Medical Record Number: Date:

MENTAL STATUS EXAM. Include the following areas as indicated: Appearance/ Attention/Attitude/Behavior, Speech (quality, quantity, flow), Mood/Affect, Suicidal and/or Homicidal Behavior/Ideation/Plan, Impulse control, Insight/judgment, Cognitive Functioning (orientation, memory, thought processes/content, ability to abstract, etc.)

Physical Appearance	( ) Appropriate	( ) Disheveled	( ) Bizarre	
Psychomotor Activity	( ) WNL	( ) Rapid	( ) Slowed	
Speech	( ) WNL ( ) Clanging	( ) Rapid	( ) Slowed	( ) Slurred
Thought Process	( ) WNL ( ) Perseverative	( ) Goal Directed ( ) Concrete	( ) Loose Assoc. ( ) Confused	( ) Tangential
Insight	( ) WNL	( ) Poor	( ) Fair	( ) Good
Judgment	( ) WNL	( ) Impulsive	( ) Impaired	
Orientation	( ) Person ( ) Delirious	( ) Place ( ) Stuperous	( ) Date ( ) Confused	( ) Alert
Memory	( ) Short Term ( ) Long Term	( ) Intact ( ) Intact	( ) Not ( ) Not	

Mood	( ) WNL ( ) Depressed ( ) Angry ( ) Irritable ( ) Confused ( ) Euphoric ( ) Anxious
Affect	( ) Congruent w/mood ( ) Appropriate ( ) Labile ( ) Flat ( ) Blunted ( ) Constricted ( ) Euphoric ( ) Anxious
Hallucinations	( ) Auditory ( ) Visual ( ) Tactile ( ) None Evident ( ) Olfactory ( ) Command ( ) Denies
Delusions	( ) None ( ) Persecutory ( ) Religious ( ) Grandiose ( ) Jealous ( ) Erotomanic
Sleep	( ) WNL ( ) Increased ( ) Decreased
Appetite	( ) WNL ( ) Increased ( ) Decreased
Suicidal	( ) Yes ( ) No ( ) Denies
Homicidal	( ) Yes ( ) No ( ) Denies

MULTI AXIAL ASSESSMENT

<u>AXIS I:</u> Clinical Disorders/Other conditions that may be a focus of clinical attention.

Diagnostic Code: DSM-name:

<u>AXIS II:</u> Personality Disorders/Mental Retardation

Diagnostic Code: DSM-name:

<u>AXIS III:</u> General Medical Conditions
ICD-9-CM Code:

<u>AXIS IV:</u>
Psychosocial/Environmental Problems

<u>AXIS V: *GAF</u>   Last Year: Present:

CRISIS INTERVENTION PLAN

Date case closed by *RCMCT: Agency(ies) referred to:
Name of Care Providers(s):   Phone:
Specialist Signature: Date:
Therapist Signature: Date:
Physician Signature: Date:
Team Leader Signature   Date:
*[Key: GAF = Global Assessment of Functioning   RCMCT = Rochester Community Mobile Team]

Psychosocial/Mental Status Exam – Demographic Info

Med. Rec. #	First Name	MI
Last Name	Address	City
State	Zip	Phone
Gender	DOB	Marital Status
Primary Language	Race	Disabilities

Cultural Identity	PCP	PCP Phone Number
Alerts	Insurance Type	Date
Time Eval. Began	Time Eval Ended	Current Living Status
Referred By	Legal Status	
Chief Complaint (2-3 words: ie Suicidal, MSE, Behavioral Issues)		

Presenting Problem/Psychosocial History

Precipitating Event/Reason for Call (reason team was called by referrer today)

Symptoms (include time frames)
- Memory
- Concentration
- Appetite
- Sleep
- Mood swings
- Energy swings
- Irritability
- Tearfulness
- Feelings of Helplessness/Hopelessness
- Suicidal/Homicidal
- Hallucinations: Auditory/Visual/Tactile/Olfactory/Command

Stressors

Health Problems	Medications	Dosages

Child Specific

- Developmental Milestones (normal/abnormal?)
- Course of Pregnancy – complications? Use of street drugs/medications, etc.
- Current Grade/process in school/Special
- Ed/Ref Education/expulsions, etc.
- Childhood Disease
- Fire Setting Behaviors
- ECO and family systems issues

Multi-Axial Assessment

Axis-I (up to 3 diagnoses)
Axis-II (up to 2 diagnoses)
Axis-III (up to 3 diagnoses)
Axis-IV (up to 4 stressors)
Axis-V GAF (1 GAF score for last year
1 GAF score for present year)

Born   Reared   #Sibling
Education

HX Abuse (sexual, physical, emotional)

Relationship Status   Children

Work History   Legal Hx/Issues

Family HX Substance Use

Family Hx Illness

Client Hx Substance Use

Name	Began	Pattern of Usage	Last Used
Alcohol			
Cannabis			
Heroin			
Cocaine			

Cigarettes – Packs Per Day

Client Hx Illness

- 1st Hospitalization

- Last Hospitalization

- Current Treatment Providers/Current Appointments

Mental Status Exam

Physical Appearance	( ) Appropriate	( ) Disheveled	( ) Bizarre	
Psychomotor Activity	( ) WNL	( ) Rapid	( ) Slowed	
Speech	( ) WNL ( ) Clanging	( ) Rapid	( ) Slowed	( ) Slurred
Thought Process	( ) WNL ( ) Perseverative	( ) Goal Directed ( ) Concrete	( ) Loose Assoc. ( ) Confused	( ) Tangential
Insight	( ) WNL	( ) Poor	( ) Fair	( ) Good
Judgment	( ) WNL	( ) Impulsive	( ) Impaired	
Orientation	( ) Person ( ) Delirious	( ) Place ( ) Stuperous	( ) Date ( ) Confused	( ) Alert
Memory	( ) Short Term ( ) Long Term	( ) Intact ( ) Intact	( ) Not ( ) Not	
Mood	( ) WNL ( ) Confused	( ) Depressed ( ) Euphoric	( ) Angry ( ) Anxious	( ) Irritable
Affect	( ) Congruent w/mood ( ) Flat ( ) Anxious	( ) Blunted	( ) Appropriate ( ) Constricted	( ) Labile ( ) Euphoric
Hallucinations	( ) Auditory ( ) Olfactory	( ) Visual ( ) Command	( ) Tactile ( ) Denies	( ) None Evident
Delusions	( ) None ( ) Grandiose	( ) Persecutory ( ) Jealous	( ) Religious ( ) Erotomanic	
Sleep	( ) WNL	( ) Increased	( ) Decreased	
Appetite	( ) WNL	( ) Increased	( ) Decreased	
Suicidal	( ) Yes	( ) No	( ) Denies	
Homicidal	( ) Yes	( ) No	( ) Denies	

Crisis Intervention Plan/Worked On the Scene:
What team did, emergency contacts, new appointments, etc.

Name of Care Providers Referred To:
Phone Number:
Agency:
Crisis Specialist:
Crisis Therapist:
Date:

Appendix F

LEGEND OF ABBREVIATIONS:
CLINICAL AND PSYCHIATRIC TERMS

abn.	abnormal	FSIQ	Full scale I.Q.
AWOL	absent without leave	HTP	House-Tree-Person Test
adol.	adolescent	HWI	healthy white infant
ACOA	Adult Children of Alcoholics	hx.	history
ACA	against clinical advice	HV	home visit
ETOH	alcohol	ILP	Independent Living Program
ACS	Alternate Care Status	indv.	Individual
ASL	American Sign Language	IEP	Individualized Education
acd.	anticipated completion date		Program
ATC	around the clock	I.Q.	Intelligence Quotient
ADHD	Attention Deficit Hyperactivity	JD	juvenile delinquent
	Disorder	J.O.	juvenile offender
ADD	Attention Deficit Disorder	KFD	Kinetic Family Drawing Test
ALOS	average length of stay	LD	learning disability
A.T.	Art Therapist	LOS	length of stay
BATA	Belief Art Therapy Assessment	MH	marital history
BG	Bender-Gestalt	MR	mentally retarded
CC	Chief Complaint	M.I.	mentally ill
CPS	Child Protective Service	n.s.	no show
COA	children of alcoholics	NLU	nonlegal union
cf	cite further	NOS	NOT OTHERWISE
CSE	Committee on Special		SPECIFIED
	Education	OT	Occupational Therapy
conf.	conference	O	Official
CON	consultation	PH	Past History
CAN	consultation as needed	PIAT	Peabody Individual
DDS	Diagnostic Drawing Series		Achievement Test
DTLA – 2	Detroit Test of Learning	PIQ	Performance I.Q.
	Aptitude	PC	phone call
dx.	diagnosis	PDR	Physician's Desk Reference
DSM-III	Diagnostic & Statistical	Post. Pl.	post-placement
	Manual of Mental Disorders	preg. couns.	pregnancy counseling
dc.	discharge	PN	progress notes
DSM III-R	DSM III-Revised	psy.	psychiatric
DSM IV R	DSM IV-Revised	pso.	psychological
EH	emotionally handicapped	RT	Residential Treatment
eval.	evaluation	R/O	rule out
fs	family session	SAMH	Severe and Multiply
fh	family history		Handicapped
fm. mtg.	family meeting	SDT	Silver Drawing Test
FT	family therapy	Sp. Ed.	Special Education
FC	foster care	S.P.	Speech Pathology
fp	foster parent	TAT	Thematic Apperception Test

TPR	therapeutic physical restraint, termination of parental rights	WAIS	Wechsler Adult Intelligence Scale
TMR	trainable mentally retarded	WISC	Wechsler Intelligence Scale for Children
tx.	treatment		
TC	treatment conference	WRAT	Wide Range Achievement Test
U	update	WNL	within normal limits
VIQ	Verbal I.Q.	WRDI	Woodcock Reading Diagnostic Inventory
VMI	visual motor integration		
WISC-R	Wechsler Intelligence Scale for Children-Revised		

Affiliations and Accreditations

AATA	American Art Therapy Association	I.C.	Interpreter Certificate
		JCAHO	Joint Commission of Accreditation of Healthcare Organizations
ACSW	Academy of Certified Social Workers		
Assoc.	Association	M.A.	Masters of Arts
B.A.	Baccalaureate Arts Degree	NCSP	Nationally Certified School Psychologist
B.S.	Baccalaureate Science Degree		
BSW	Bachelor of Social Work	RSC	Reverse Skills Certificate
EPAB	Education Program Approval Board (of AATA)	SUNY	State University of New York
		T.C.	Translator Certificate
GED	General Education Diploma/ High School Equivalency	UYA	University Year of Action

General Terms and Miscellaneous

AWOL	absent without leave	bio.	biological, birth
Add.	addendum	B/W	biracial
adj.	adjustment	B/D	birth date
adol.	adolescent	b-day	birthday
ETOH	alcohol	Bl. or B	black
AKA	also known as	bldg.	building
ASL	American Sign Language	per	by way of
amt.	amount	cal.	calorie
ans.	answer	Cauc.	Caucasian
apt.	apartment	ctr.	center
app.	application	CNY	Central New York
appt.	appointment	chn	children
ASAP	as soon as possible	cf	cite further
ad. lib.	as desired	CSE	Committee on Special Education
Assoc.	Association		
A.V.	audio visual	comm.	communication
Ave.	avenue	conf.	conference
ALOS	average length of stay	CAN	consultation as needed
am	before noon	CON	consultation
a	before	cont.'d	continued
btwn.	between	ct.	court

DOB	date of birth	N/A	not applicable
D.C.	daycare	OV	office visit
DAT	Diagnostic Assessment Team	O	official
dc	discharge	pkg.	package
D/C	discontinue	pg.	page
dist.	district	pt.	patient
div.	divorce	PC	phone call
EBT	early bedtime	PSE	Pigeon Signed English
educ.	education	P.S.	postscript
ER	emergency room	K	Potassium
ED	Emergency Department	PROB(s)	problems
etc.	etcetera, and so on	prog.	program
eval.	evaluation	PN	progress notes
fh	family history	rec'd	received
F. Ct.	Family Court	rec.	recommendation
e.g.	for example	Rec.	Recreation
F	Forman	ref.	reference
F.H.	foster home	re:	regarding
freq.	frequent	rel.	relationship
f.t.	full-time	rev.	review
gr.	grain	r	right
grp.	group	sch.	school
HS	high school	sect	section
HILP	Home Improvement Loan Program	Sr.	senior
		SSD	Social Security Disability
Hmkr.	homemaker	St.	street
hosp.	hospital	i.e.	such as, to wit, specifically, that is
stat	immediately		
indv.	individual	supv.	supervision
info.	information	SSI	Supplemental Security Income
info. mtg.	information meeting	Tbsp.	tablespoon
int.	international	tsp.	teaspoon
jr.	junior	TDD	Telecommunication Device for the Deaf
K.M.	Key Math		
l	left	TTY	Teletype Telephone
mgmt.	management	TV	television
MCE	Manually Coded English	tx	treatment
MH	marital history	TC	treatment conference
MA	Medicaid	U	university
mtg.	meeting	unk.	unknown
msg.	message	vac.	vacation
viz.	namely	voc.	vocational
nat.	natural	wk.	week
neg.	negative	c	with
N.Y.S.	New York State	w/	with
N.Y.C.	New York City	S	without
n.s.	no show	w/o	without
NLU	nonlegal union	WIN	Work Incentive
norm.	normal	y/o	years old

Medical and Physical Terms

abd	abdomen, abdominal	eval.	evaluation
abn.	abnormal	qod	every other day
AIDS	Acquired Immune Deficiency Syndrome	qhs	every nigh
		qh	every hour
pc	after meals	q.	every
ETOH	alcohol	q 4h	every 4 hours
ATC	around the clock	qd	everyday
ad. lib.	as desired	FBS	fasting blood sugar
as fol.	as tolerated	FB	foreign body
prn	as necessary	q.i.d.	four times a day
hs	at bedtime	GI	gastrointestinal
ac	before meals	GU	genitor-urinary
bio.	biological, birth	GTT	glucose tolerance test
b.c.p.	birth control pills	GC	gonorrhea
BP	blood pressure	GYN	gynecology
BC/BS	Blue Cross Blue Shield	HWI	healthy white infant
OU	both eyes	HD	hearing distance
AU	both ears	H.I.	hearing impaired
BM	bowel movement	ht.	height
p.o.	by mouth	Hep-A	Hepatitis-A
CDC	calculated day of treatment	Hep-B	Hepatitis-B
cap	capsule	hosp.	hospital
CPR	cardiopulmonary resuscitation	H.I.V.	human immunodeficiency virus
CNS	central nervous system		
CP	Cerebral Palsy	sos	if necessary
C-section	caesarean section	stat	immediately
CC	chief complaint	IM	intramuscular
CBS	chronic brain syndrome	IV	intravenous
CBC	complete blood count	LMP	last menstrual period
CAT Scan	Computerized Axial Tomography Scan	AS	left ear
		OS	left eye
CT Scan	Computerized Tomography Scan	LPN	Licensed Practical Nurse
		LOM	limitation of motion
CAN	consultation as needed	LOC	loss of consciousness
cc	cubic centimeter	MRI Scan	Magnetic Resonance Imaging
DOB	date of birth	med.	medical
dx.	diagnosis	M.D.	medical doctor
D/C	discontinue	meds.	medication
Dr.	doctor	MI	myocardial infarction
dsg.	dressing	neg.	negative
gtt(s).	drops	NB	newborn
ENT	ear, nose and throat	NKA	no known allergies
EEG	electroencephalogram	norm.	normal
EKG	electrocardiogram	NPO	nothing by mouth
ER	emergency room	OB	obstetrics
ED	Emergency Department	OV	office visit
EDC	estimated date of confinement	OCP	oral contraceptive pills

OBS	Organic Brain Syndrome	SOB	shortness of breath
ortho.	orthopedics	strep	streptococcus
Pap	Papanicolaou	Tbsp.	tablespoon
PH	past history	tab.	tablet
path	pathology	tsp.	teaspoon
pt.	patient	T.	temperature
Ped.	Pediatrician	t.i.d.	three times a day
PID	pelvic inflammatory disease	TC	throat culture
PNS	peripheral nervous system	tx.	treatment
PKU	Phenylketonuria	b.i.d.	twice a day
PT	Physical Therapy, physical therapist	US	ultrasound
		unk.	unknown
P.A.	Physician's Assistant	URI	upper respiratory infection
PDR	Physician's Desk Reference	UTI	urinary tract infection
PMS	pre-menstrual syndrome	vag.	Vaginal
Rx.	prescription	VD	venereal disease
PMP	previous menstrual period	VDRL	venereal disease research laboratory
P	pulse		
RBC	red blood count	VA	visual acuity
R.N.	Registered Nurse	Wt.	weight
R	respiration	WD	well developed
Rh Pos	rhesus factor positive	WN	well nourished
Rh Neg	rhesus factor negative	WBC	white blood count
AD	right hear	c gl.	with glasses
OD	right eye	WNL	within normal limits
RLQ	right lower quadrant	s gl.	without glasses
rt	right	S	without
R/O	rule out	y/o	years old
STD	sexually transmitted disease		

Legal Terms

ACD	Adjournment in Contemplation of Dismissal	L	L-review
		LG	Law Guardian
AKA	also known as	PINS	Persons in Need of Supervision
ct.	court	I-600	Petition to classify orphan as immediate relative
F. Ct.	Family Court		
H of J	Hall of Justice	P.O.	Probation Officer
J.O.	Juvenile Offender	PL	Public Law
JD	Juvenile Delinquent	Y.O.	Youthful Offender
K	K-review		

Internal HCC Names and Terms

ADL	Activities of Daily Living	AMC	All My Children
AOBH	Agency Operated Boarding Home	A.I .Y	Alternatives for Independent Youth
Alex.	Alexander Group Home	Arnt.	Arnett Group Home

BGR	B. Group Runner		IFS	Intensive Family Support Program
Bau.	Bausch Cottage		Lab.	Laburnum Group Home
C.S.	Campus School		LSW BOCES	Livingston, Steuben, Wyoming Co. BOCES
CCW	Child Care Worker		MDR	Multidisciplinary Review
CT	Communication Therapy		NSD	Non-Secure Detention
CBGC	Community Based Group Care		NH	Northaven
DACT	Dads and Children Together		OPT	Opportunities for Pregnant & Parenting Teens
D.T.	Day Treatment		Preg. Couns.	Pregnancy Counseling
Div.	Diversion		Prev.	Preventive
EBT	Early Bedtime		PSO	Professional Staff Organization
Emerg. Prog.	Emergency Program		QA/EH	Quality Assurance/ Environmental Health
FV	Fairview Cottage		Rec.	Recreation
FRS	Family Resource Specialist		RTC	Residential Treatment Center
FPS	Family Preservation Service		RT	Residential Treatment
FLE	Family Life Education		RTF	Residential Treatment Facility
GH	Group Home		RTFC	Rochester Therapeutic Foster Care
H.I.	Hearing Impaired		ST	Sociotherapist
HDT	Henrietta Day Treatment		SS	Sunnyside Cottage
HCC	Hillside Children's Center		STFC	Syracuse Therapeutic Foster Care
HIBS	Hillside Intensive Homebased Services		TPR	Therapeutic Physical Restraint
Hill Cap	Hillside Chemical Abuse Program		TFC	Therapeutic Foster Care
HIFS	Hillside Intensive Family Service Program		UR	Utilization Review
HSP	Human Sexuality Program		VF	Visiting Friend
Hutch	Hutchison Cottage		VVF	Volunteer Visiting Friend
IHD	In-Home Diversion		WS	Woodside Cottage
I.R.	Incident Report			
ILP	Independent Living Program			
ITK	Intake			

DSS Terms

CID	Case Initiation Date		MCDSS	Monroe County Department of Social Services
CIN	Case Identification Number		Neg.	Neglect
CPS	Child Protective Service		PPG	Permanency Planning Goal
DSS	Department of Social Services		I-600	Petition to classify orphan as immediate relative
dist.	District		P.A.	Plan Amendment
FCI	Foster Care Intake		PA	Public Assistance
fp	foster parent		RASPR	Reassessment & Service Plan Review
FC	Foster Care		SSD	Social Security Disability
F.H.	Foster Home		SSA	Social Security Administration
I.M.	Income Maintenance		SCR	State Central Registry
IASP	Initial Assessment and Service Plan		SSI	Supplemental Security Income
K	K-review		TPR	termination of parental rights
L	L-review			
MA	Medicaid			

| UCR | Uniform Case Record | UR | Utilization Review |
| UR/TM | Utilization Review/Treatment Monitoring | WIC | Women, Infant, Children Nutrition Program |

Organizations and Agencies

AATA	American Art Therapy Association	MCDSS	Monroe County Department of Social Services
ABC	Action for a Better Community	MCH	Monroe Community Hospital
APPS	Adolescent Pregnancy & Parenting Service	MDC	Monroe Developmental Center
AA	Alcoholics Anonymous	MCCC	Monroe County Children's Center
ABW	Alternatives for Battered Women	MCC	Monroe Community College
AJHC	Anthony Jordon Health Center	N.A.	Narcotic Anonymous
ARC	Association for Retarded Citizens	NTID	National Technical Institute for the Deaf
BC/BS	Blue Cross/Blue Shield	OVS	Office of Volunteer Services
Bd of Ed.	Board of Education	OMH	Office of Mental Health
CFC	Catholic Family Center	VESID	Office of Vocational & Educational Services for Individuals with Disabilities
CSE	Committee on Special Education		
CPY	Community Partners for Youth	P.P.	Planned Parenthood
CETA	Concentrated Employment Training Act	RTS	Regional Transit System
		RID	Registry of Interpreters for the Deaf
CAP	Council of Adoptive Parents		
CCC	Crestwood Children's Center	RSD	Rochester School for the Deaf
DSS	Department of Social Services	RMHC	Rochester Mental Health Center
DFY	Division for Youth		
ECC	Eastside Community Center	RPC	Rochester Psychiatric Center
EOC	Educational Opportunity Center	RIT	Rochester Institute of Technology
EPC	Elmira Psychiatric Center	RHA	Rochester Housing Authority
FSR	Family Services of Rochester	RGE	Rochester Gas & Electric
FACIT	Family Crisis Intervention Team	RPD	Rochester Police Department
		RGH	Rochester General Hospital
GMHC	Genesee Mental Health Center	RCSD	Rochester City School District
GA	Gustavus Adolphus	RAMP	Rochester Adolescent Maternity Program
HPC	Hutchings Psychiatric Center		
IBERO	Ibero-American Action League	SSA	Social Security Administration
		S.E.D.	State Education Department
INS	Immigration and Naturalization Service	SMH	Strong Memorial Hospital
		TFT	Teen Family Team
IAG	International Adoption Group (of CAP)	TAPSS	Teenage Parent Support Services
MHIS	Mental Health Information Service	T.G.H.	The Genesee Hospital
		TASA	Therapeutic Alternatives for Sexual Abuse
MVCPC	Mohawk Valley Children's Psychiatric Center		

WAFRC	Webster Avenue Family Resource Center	WIN	Work Incentive
WNYCPC	Western New York Children's Psychiatric Center	YMCA	Young Women's Christian Association
WMMH	Western Monroe Mental Health	Yo. Mo's Pgrm. YMCA	Young Mother's Program Young Men's Christian Association

Family Members and Race

B/W	bi-racial	f.o.b.	father of baby
b.f.	boyfriend	g. f.	girlfriend
bro.	brother	g.fa.	grandfather
Cauc.	Caucasian	g.mo.	grandmother
chn.	Children	Hisp.	Hispanic
dau.	Daughter	HV	home visit
div.	divorce	Hmkr.	homemaker
fs	family session	MH	marital history
FT	family therapy	mo.	mother
fm.mtg.	family meeting	M/M	Mr. and Mrs.
fh	family history	NB	newborn
fam.	family	NLU	nonlegal union
fam. of O or FOO	family of origin	Sr. sib.	senior sibling
Home FS	Family Session (Treatment) at Home	t.m. t.f.	teen mother teen father
fa.	father		

Titles

ACSW	Academy of Certified Social Workers	Dir. Ph.D.	Director Doctor of Philosophy
ACCW	Accredited Child Care Worker	Ed. Spec.	Educational Specialist
ART	Accredited Record Technician	Exec.	Executive
ACOA	Adult Children of Alcoholics	FRS	Family Resource Specialist
A.T.R.	Art Therapist Registered	HSL	Human Sexuality Leader
A.T.R.–B.C. or ATR-BC	Art Therapist Registered, Board Certified	ILS LPN	Independent Living Specialist Licensed Practical Nurse
A.A.	Associate of Arts Degree	M.S.	Master of Science
CTA	Certified Teaching Assistant	M.S.W.	Master of Social Work
CTRS	Certified Therapeutic Recreation Specialist	M.D. MTBC	Medical Doctor Music Therapist, Board Certified
CSW	Certified Social Worker		
CRT	Certified Recreation Therapist	Ped.	Pediatrician
CAC	Certified Alcohol Counselor	PT	Physical Therapist
CCW	Child Care Worker	PCCW	Primary Child Care Worker
COA	Children of Alcoholics	P.O.	Probation Officer
CHN	Community Health Nurse	Prog. Aide	Program Aide
CSC	Comprehensive Skills Certificate (Interpreter)	P.S.W. Rec. T.	Psychiatric Social Worker Recreation Therapist

R.N.	Registered Nurse	sup.	supervisor
RS	Resource Volunteer	T.A.	Teacher's Assistant
R.T.	Resource Teacher	UV	Unit Volunteer
SW	Social Worker	VF	Visiting Friend
ST	Sociotherapist	VVF	Volunteer Visiting Friend
SET	Special Education Teacher	Vol.	Volunteer
S.T.	Speech Therapist	Y.O.	Youthful Offender

Religions

AG	Assembly of God	LU	Lutheran
BH	Bahai	ME	Methodist
BA	Baptist	LD	Mormon
BR	Brethren	NP	No Preference
BU	Buddhist	OR	Orthodox
RC	Catholic	OT	Other
CS	Christian Science	PT	Pentecostal
ND	Christian (nondenominational)	UP	Presbyterian
CG	Congregational	PR	Protestant
DC	Disciples of Christ	RF	Reformed
EP	Episcopal	SD	Seventh Day Adventist
ER	Evangelical and Reformed	FR	Soc. Of Friends Quakers
GO	Greek Orthodox	UN	Unitarian
HI	Hindu	CC	United Church of Christ
IS	Islam	UV	Universalist
JU	Jewish	WS	Wesleyan

Measurements and Time

p	after	freq.	frequent
pm	afternoon	f.t.	full time
amt.	amount	gm.	gram
ASAP	as soon as possible	hrs.	hours
ALOS	average length of stay	in.	inches
a	before	LOS	length of stay
am	before noon	max.	maximum
cal.	calorie	mg.	milligram
ctr.	center	ml.	milliliter
C	Centigrade	mm.	millimeter
cm.	centimeter	min.	minimum
ca.	circa, about	mo.	month
cont.'d.	continued	oz.	ounce
q.	every	lb.	pound
qd	everyday	PLOS	projected length of stay
F	Fahrenheit	wk.	week
ft.	feet	y/o	years old

Symbols

@	at	#	number
↑	elevated	#1, #2, etc.	one, two, etc.
♀	female	+	plus
>	greater than	ψ	psychologist
<	less than	X	times
↓	reduced	H_2O	water
♂	male	=	equal
–	minus	1:1	one to one

ABBREVIATIONS

abd.	Abdomen, abdominal	ARC	Association for Retarded Citizens
AWOL	Absent without leave		
ACSW	Academy of Certified Social Workers	Attn.	Attention
		ADD	Attention deficit disorder
AI	Acute intoxication	ADHD	Attention deficit hyperactivity disorder
AOM	Acute Otitus Media		
ACD	Adjournment in Contemplation of Dismissal	AIDS	Acquired Immune Deficiency Syndrome
ASFA	Adoption and Safe Family Act	Aug.	August
ACOA	Adult Children of Alcoholics	Ave.	Avenue
APS	Adult Protective Services	BA	Bachelor of Arts
p	After	BS	Bachelor of Science
ASW	Aftercare Social Worker	BSN	Bachelor of Science in Nursing
P.M.	Afternoon	BSW	Bachelor of Social Work
AMA	Against Medical Advice	BV	Bacterial Vaginosis
A.E.	Age Equivalent	b/c	Because
ETOH	Alcohol	hs.	Bedtime (hour of sleep)
AA	Alcoholics Anonymous	a	Before
A.C.D.	Alternate Care Determination	A.M.	Before noon
AHIMA	American Health Information Management Association	beh.	Behaviors
		Bender	Bender-Gestalt
amt.	Amount	BOM	Bilatecal Otitis Media
ans.	Answer	bio.	Biological, birth
&	And	BCP	Birth Control Pills
apt./Apt.	Apartment	b.d.	Birth date
appt.	Appointment	Blk.	Black
	Approximate	bo.	Black out
Apr.	April	BAC	Blood Alcohol Content
prn.	As necessary	BG	Blood Glucose
ASAP	As soon as possible	BP	Blood pressure
Ass't.	Assistant	BC/BS	Blue Cross/Blue Shield
ADGH	Assistant Director of Group Home	Bl.Ch.	Blue Choice
		BOE	Board of Education
Assoc.	Associate	O.U.	Both eyes

BM	Bowel Movement	CCC	Crestwood Children's Center
bro.	Brother	CIS	Crisis Intervention Specialist
po	By mouth	cc.	Cubic centimeter
CA	Cancer	C&S	Culture and sensitivity
cap.	Capsule	DU	Daily use of chemicals
Cath.	Catholic	dob	Date of birth
CFC	Catholic Family Center	dop.	Date of placement
W	Caucasian	dau.	Daughter
ctr.	Center	Day Tx	Day Treatment
C	Centigrade	Dec.	December
cm.	Centimeter	db	Decibels
CASAC	Certified Alcohol and	DDS	Dentist
	Substance Abuse Counselor	DSS	Department of Social Services
C.T.R.S.	Certified Therapeutic	DD	Developmental Disability
	Recreation Specialist	VMI	Developmental test of
CRC	Certified Rehabilitation		Visual Motor Integration
	Counselor	Dx	Diagnosis
CSW	Certified Social Worker	BRAT	Diet for Diarrhea (bananas,
CSW-R	Certified Social Worker		rice, applesauce, toast)
	with R#	diff.	Difficult
c/s	Caesarean section	Dir.	Director
or c-section		DOE	Director of Education
▲	Change	DGH	Director of Group Homes
ca	Chemically abusive	DPS	Director of Preventive Services
CD	Chemically dependent	DRT	Director of Residential
CCW	Child Care Worker		Treatment
COA	Child of Alcoholic	d/c	Discharge
CPA	Child Protective Service	d/s	Discharge Summary
CI	Chronic intoxication	DHD	Discovery Huther Doyle
CSM	Circulation, sensation,	dist.	District
	movement	DA	District Attorney
CD	Clinical Director	DFY	Division for Youth
CELF	Clinical Evaluation of	div.	Divorce
	Language Fundamentals	Dr.	Doctor
CSO	Clinical Staff Organization	Ed.D.	Doctor of Education
codep.	Co-dependent	D.O.	Doctor of Osteopathy
CSE	Committee on Special Ed	Ph.D.	Doctor of Philosophy
CHN	Community Health Network	Psy.D.	Doctor of Psychology
CR	Community Residence	gtts.	Drop(s)
c/o	Complains of	DOC	Drug of Choice
CBC	Complete Blood Count	D.S.D.	Dry sterile dressing
CBCcdiff.	Complete Blood Count with	d/t	Due to
	Differential	Eat.Dis.	Eating Disorder
conf.	Conference	EMR	Educable Mentally Retarded
CPM	Continue Present Management	educ.	Education
CDT	Continuing Day Treatment	ed voc coord	Educational-vocational
CAP	Council on Adoptive Parents		coordinator
ct	Court	EKG ECG	Electrocardiogram
CAC	Credentialed Alcoholism	EEG	Electroencephalogram
	Counselor	Emerg.	Emergency

E.R.	Emergency Room	gr.fa.	Grandfather
E.D.	Emotionally Disturbed	gr.mo.	Grandmother
EH	Emotionally handicapped	gp.	Group
EEU	Episodic use of chemicals	GH	Group Home
etc.	Etcetera, and so on	GA	Gustavas Adolphus
Eval.	Evaluation	GYN	Gynecology
q.d.	Every day	HEC	Halpern Education Center
q.4h.	Every four hours	HO	Health Office
q.h.	Every hour	ht.	Height
q.o.d.	Every other day	HS	High School
EU	Experimental use of chemicals	HCC	Hillside Children's Center
E(ENT)	Eye, ear, nose, throat	Hisp.	Hispanic
F	Fahrenheit	Hx	History
fm.	Family	HILP	Home Improvement Loan
Fm.Ct.	Family court		Program
FACIT	Family Crisis Intervention	Hmkr.	Homemaker
	Team	HV	Home visit
fm.mtg.	Family meeting	hosp.	Hospital
FSR	Family Service of Rochester	hr or o	Hour
FT	Family therapy	HE	Human Ecology
fa	Father	HIV (+/−)	Human Immunodeficiency
FOB	Father of Baby		Virus (positive or negative)
Feb.	February	STAT	Immediate
ft.	Feet	in.	Inches
Ms.	Female title used without	ILS	Independent Life Skills
	regard to marital status	ind	Individual
FU	First Use of Drugs	IEP	Individual Education Program
F/U	Follow-up	IA	Industrial Arts
e.g.	For example	info.	Information
F.B.	Foreign body	info.mtg.	Information Meeting
FCI	Foster Care Intake	inj.	Injection
F.H.	Foster Home	IQ	Intelligence Quotient
FP	Foster Parent	IFSP	Intensive Family Support
q.i.d.	Four times a day		Program
fx	Fracture	IOP	Intensive Outpatient Program
f.g.p.	Fraternal grandparents	intern	Intern student
FDI	Freedom from Distractibility	Int.	International
	Index	I.M.	Intramuscular
FSIQ	Full Scale Intelligence	IV	Intravenous
	Quotient	IPRT	Intensive Psychiatric
G.I.	Gastrointestinal		Rehabilitation Treatment
GED	General education diploma	Jan.	January
	(High School Equivalency)	JTPA	Job Training Partnership Act
GMHC	Genesee Mental Health Center	JCAHO	Joint Commission on
G.U.	Genito-urinary		Accreditation of Healthcare
Gr.	Grade		Organizations
GC	Grade Content	JHS	Junior High School
GE	Grade Equivalent	JD	Juvenile Delinquent
GL	Grade level	K-TEA	Kaufman Test of Educational
GM	Gram		Ability

lab	Laboratory	misc.	Miscellaneous
LMP	Last Menstrual Period	MCDSS	Monroe County Department of Social Services
LG	Law guardian		
LD	Learning disability/learning disabled	MDC	Monroe Developmental Center
L	Left	mo.	Month
O.S.	Left eye	Mo	Mother
LLQ	Left lower quadrant	M/M	Mr. and Mrs.
LUQ	Left upper quadrant	NA	Narcotics Anonymous
LPN	Licensed Practical Nurse	nat.	Natural
LST	Life Skills Trainer	–	Negative
LEA	Local education authority	N.Y.	New York
Ic	Loss of control over alcohol or chemical use	NYC	New York City
		NYS	New York State
mgr.	Manager	NAD	No Acute Distress
manage.	Management	NKDA	No Known Drug Allergies
Mar.	March	N/S	No show
THC	Marijuana	NG	Non-Graded
Mrs.	Married Women	NSD	Non-Secure Detention
MA	Master of Arts	NSD	Normal Spontaneous Delivery
M.Ed.	Master of Education	N/A	Not applicable
MPA	Master of Public Administration	NOS	Not otherwise specified
		NPO	Nothing by mouth
MS	Master of Science	Nov.	November
MSSW	Matter of Science and Social Work	NP	Nurse Practitioner
		OB/GYN	Obstetrician/gynecologist
MSEC	Master of Science Educational Counseling	O.T.	Occupational Therapy
		Oct.	October
MS.Ed.	Master of Science in Education	OASAS	Office of Alcohol/Substance Abuse Service
MSSA	Master of Social Science and Administration	OMH	Office of Mental Health
		OVR	Office of Vocational Rehabilitation
MSW	Master of Social Work		
m.gr.p.	Maternal grandparents	OV	Office Visit
MDD	Maximum Daily Dose	OCDSS	Onondaga County Department of Social Services
MA	Medicaid		
med	Medical	oz.	Ounce
ME	Medicare	OOP	Out of Program
MD	Medical Doctor	OOR	Out of Routine
ME	Medical Examiner	OA	Overeaters Anonymous
mtg.	Meeting	PIAT	Peabody Individual Achievement Test
MH	Mental Health		
MI	Mental Illness	Pap Smear	Papanicolaou
MR	Mental Retardation	PRCD	Park Ridge Chemical Dependency
msg.	Message		
mg.	Milligram	PRH	Park Ridge Hospital
ml.	Milliliter	PHP	Partial Hospitalization Program
mm.	Millimeter		
MMPI	Minnesota Multi-phasic Personality Inventory	PPVT	Peabody Picture Vocabulary Test
mm.	Minute		

Ped.	Pediatrician	RRA	Registered Record
P.I.D.	Pelvic Inflammatory Disease		Administrator
POI	Perceptual Organization Index	rel.	Relapse
PIQ	Performance Intelligence	RC	Residential Counselor
	Quotient	RT	Residential Treatment
PINS/T	Person in Need of	RTC	Residential Treatment Center
	Supervision/Truancy	RTF	Residential Treatment Facility
PINS/U	Person in Need of	Resp.	Respiration
	Supervision/Ungovernable	RICE	Rest, Ice, compression,
Phys.	Physical		elevation
P.Ed.	Physical Education	Rev.	Reverend
P.E.	Physical Exam	retol.	Reverse tolerance
P.T.	Physical Therapy	rev.	Review
P.A.	Physician's Assistant	®	Right
Pls.	Please	O.D.	Right eye
pt.	Point	RLQ	Right lower quadrant
PCU	Poly Chemical Use	RUQ	Right upper quadrant
+	Positive	Rd.	Road
PP	Postpartum	Roch.	Rochester
lb.	Pound	RCSD	Rochester City School District
PC	Preferred Care	RGE	Rochester Gas and Electric
PT	Pregnancy Test	RGH	Rochester General Hospital
PCT	Preliminary Competency Test	RIT	Rochester Institute of
Rx	Prescription		Technology
PCP	Primary Care Physician	RMHC	Rochester Mental Health
l ther	Primary Therapist		Center
PO	Probation Officer	RPD	Rochester Police Department
PSI	Processing Speed Index	RPC	Rochester Psychiatric Center
prog.	Program	RRC	Rochester Rehabilitation
PEU	Progressive excessive use		Center
Prot.	Protestant	RSD	Rochester School for the Deaf
Y eval	Psychiatric Evaluation	sch.	School
psych.	Psychological	SY	School year
P.S. (eval)	Psychosocial Evaluation	2°	Secondary
PA	Public Assistance	ESR	Sedimentation rate
PD	Public Defender	SASW	Senior Aftercare Social
PL	Public Law		Worker
P	Pulse	Sr.Conn	Senior Connection
PERLA	Pupils equally reactive to	SHS	Senior High School
	light accommodation	S.T.S.S.W.	Senior Transitional Services
R.O.M.	Range of motion		Social Worker
rec'd	Received	Sept.	September
rec.	Recommendation	srvc.	Service
Rec.	Recreation	STD(s)	Sexually Transmitted
Rec. T.	Recreation Therapist		Disease(s)
ref.	Reference	SAQ	Short are quads
re:	Regarding	S.O.B.	Shortness of breath
RCT	Regents Competency Test	sib.	Sibling
RTS	Regional Transit System	SR	Sick Routine
RN	Registered Nurse	SER	Significant Event Report

SO	Significant Other	T.S.S.W.	Transitional Services Social Worker
S/S	Signs and symptoms		
sm.	Small	TBI	Traumatic Brain Injury
SSA	Social Security Administration	Tx	Treatment
SSD	Social Security Disability	TB	Tuberculosis
SSI	Social Security Income	b.i.d.	Twice a day
SS#	Social Security Number	UCR	Uniform Case Record
SW	Social Worker	U of R	University of Rochester
SU	Solitary use of Chemicals	unk.	Unknown
Sp Ed	Special Education	UI	Untoward Incident
Ed.S.	Specialist in Education	URI	Upper Respiratory Infection
spec.	Specimen	UTI	Urinary Tract Infection
Sp.Ther.	Speech Therapist	UR	Utilization Review
St.	State	vag.	Vaginal
SJV	St. Joseph's Villa	VCI	Verbal comprehension Index
SMH	St Mary' Hospital	VIQ	Verbal Intelligence Quotient
SED	State Education Department	VA	Veterans Administration
SUNY	State University of New York	VF	Visiting Friend
s/p	Status Post	Voc. Ed	Vocational Education
SLR	Straight leg rises	VESID	Vocational and Education Services For Individuals w/Disabilities
st.	Street		
strep	Streptococcus		
SMH	Strong Memorial Hospital	vol.	Volunteer
s.c.	Subcutaneous	WCDSS	Wayne County Department of Social Services
SLR	Supervised Independent Living Program	WAIS-III	Wechsler Adult Intelligence Scale-3rd Edition
supv.	Supervision		
Supv.	Supervisor	WIAT	Wechsler Individual Achievement Test
T	Tablespoon		
tab	Tablet	WAIS-R	Wechsler Intelligence Scale for Adults Revised
TA	Teaching Assistant Teacher's Aide	WISC-Ill	Wechsler Intelligence Scale for Children-3rd Edition
tsp.	Teaspoon		
TC	Telephone call	WISC-R	Wechsler Intelligence Scale for Children Revised
Temp.	Temperature		
T.P.R.	Temperature, pulse, respiration	WPPSI-R	Wechsler Preschool and Primary Scale of Intelligence-Revised
T.A	Temporary Assistant		
VMI	The Beery Developmental Test of Visual-Motor Integration		
TAT	Thematic Apperception Test	Wk	Week
t.i.d.	Three times a day	W/E	Weekend
T.C.	Throat Culture	WCC	Well child check
T.O.	Time Out	wt.	Weight
i.e.	To wit, specifically, that is, such as, all inclusive	c or w/	With
		W.N.L's	Within normal limits
Tol.	Tolerance	s or w/o	Without
TD	Total Dose	WRMT	Woodcock Reading Mastery Test
TMR	Trainable mentally retarded	WIC	Women, Infants, Children Nutrition Program
T.S.	Transitional Services		

WIN	Work Incentive	$=$	equal to
WMI	Working Memory Index	♀	female
yr.	Year	$>$	greater than
yrs.	Years	H_20_2	Hydrogen Peroxide
y.o	Year old	↑	Increased
YMCA	Young Men's Christian Association	$<$	less than
		↓	lowered
YWCA	Young Women's Christian Association	♂	male
		–	minus
Y.E.S.	Youth Emergency Service	#	number
Y.O.U.	Youth Opportunity Unit	O_2	Oxygen
$\approx$	about, approximately	%	percent
$+$	and	% tile	percentile
@	at	$+$	plus
$C0_2$	Carbon Dioxide	x	times
↓	decreased	H_2O	water
↑	elevated		

Appendix G

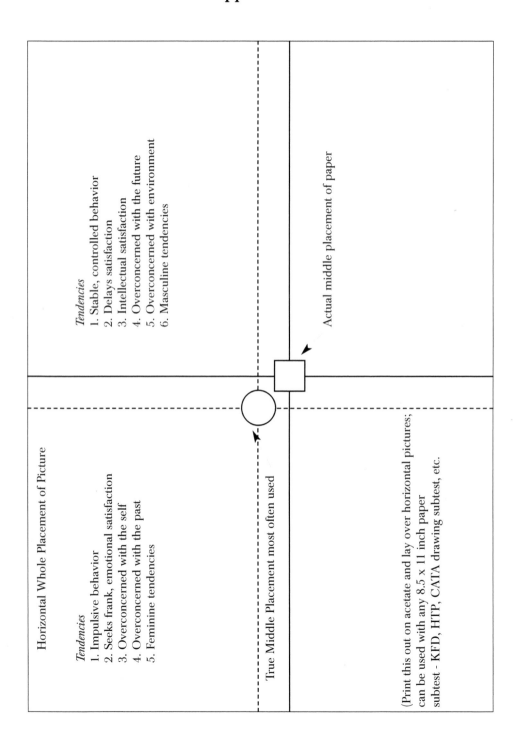

Horizontal Whole Placement of Picture

Tendencies
1. Impulsive behavior
2. Seeks frank, emotional satisfaction
3. Overconcerned with the self
4. Overconcerned with the past
5. Feminine tendencies

Tendencies
1. Stable, controlled behavior
2. Delays satisfaction
3. Intellectual satisfaction
4. Overconcerned with the future
5. Overconcerned with environment
6. Masculine tendencies

Actual middle placement of paper

True Middle Placement most often used

(Print this out on acetate and lay over horizontal pictures; can be used with any 8.5 x 11 inch paper subtest - KFD, HTP, CATA drawing subtest, etc.

Tree or Vertical Placement of Whole

Quadrant of Past Functioning

Quadrant of Present Functioning

Quadrant of Never Was Regression

(Print this out on acetate and lay over horizontal pictures; can be used with any 8.5 x 11 inch paper subtest - KFD, HTP, CATA drawing subtest, etc.

REFERENCES

Anschela, D. J., Dolceb, S., Schwartzmanc, A., & Fishera, R. S. (2005). A blinded pilot study of artwork in a comprehensive epilepsy center population. *Epilepsy & Behavior, 6,* 196–202.

Ashbrook, J. B. (1971). *Become community.* Valley Forge, Pennsylvania: Judson Press.

Bender, L. (1938). *A Visual Motor Gestalt Test and Its Clinical Use.* American Orthopsychiatric Association, Research Monographs (No. 3). New York: American Orthopsychiatric Association.

Betts, D. J. (2003). Developing a projective drawing test: Experiences with the Face Stimulus Assessment (FSA). *Art Therapy: Journal of the American Art Therapy Association, 20*(2), 77–82.

Betts, D. J. (2004). Face Stimulus Assessment (FSA): Guidelines. Unpublished handout provided for ATR 522, Nazareth College, Rochester, NY.

Betts, D. J. (2005). *A systematic analysis of art therapy assessment and rating instrument literature.* [Online]. Available: http://www.art-therapy.us/assessment.html.

Betts, D. J. (2008). Face Stimulus Assessment (FSA) guidelines. Unpublished guidebook. Tallahassee, FL: Author.

Brannigan, G. C., & Decker, S. L. (2003). *Bender Gestalt II Second Edition.* Itasca, IL: Riverside Publishing Co.

Brooke, S. L. (2004). *Tools of the trade: A therapist's guide to art therapy assessments* (2nd ed.). Springfield, IL: Charles C Thomas Publisher,

Buck, J. N. (1966). *The House-Tree-Person Technique: Revised manual.* Beverly Hills, CA: Western Psychological Services.

Burns, R. C., & Kaufman, S. H. (1972). *Actions, styles and symbols in Kinetic Family Drawings (K-F-D): An interpretive manual.* New York: Brunner/Mazel.

Cheyne-King, S. E. (1990). Effects of brain injury on visual perception and art production. *The Arts in Psychotherapy, 17,* 69–74.

Cohen, F. W., & Phelps, R. E. (1985). Incest Markers in Children's Art Work. *The Arts in Psychotherapy, 12,* 265–283.

DiLeo, J. H. (1970). *Young children and their drawings.* New York, NY: Brunner/Mazel.

Dearing, T. (1983). *God and healing of the mind: A spiritual guide to mental health.* South Plainfield, NJ: Bridge Publications.

Dombeck, M., & Karl, J. (1987). Spiritual issues in mental health. *Journal of Religion & Health.* Fall, Vol. 26 (3): 183–197.

Fowler, J. W. (1981). *Stages of faith: The psychology of human development and the quest for meaning.* San Francisco: Harper.

Frank, J. D., & Frank, J. B. (1991). *Persuasion and healing: A comparative study of psychotherapy.* 3rd Edition, Baltimore, MD: Johns H opkins University Press.

Freud's stages of psychosexual development: The anal stage. [Online]. Available: http://psychology. about.com/od/theoriesofpersonality/ss/psychosexualdev_3.html

Gantt, L., & Tabone, C. (1998). *Formal Elements Art Therapy Scale: The rating manual.* Morgantown, WV: Gargoyle Press.

Gantt, L. (2001). The Formal Elements Art Therapy Scale: A measurement system for global variables in art. *Art Therapy: Journal of the American Art Therapy Association, 18* (1), 50–55.

Griffiths, R. (1935). *A study of imagination in early childhood.* London: Kegan, Paul, Trench, Trubner & Co.

Guerin, P., & Pendagast, E. (1976). Evaluation of family system and genogram (p. 450–464). In Guerin, P. J. (Ed.), *Family therapy: Theory and practice.* New York: Gardner Press.

Hall, J. (1979). *Dictionary of subjects and symbols in art.* New York, NY: Harper & Row.

Hamilton, M., & Betts, D. (2008). Developing a standardized rating system for the Face Stimulus Assessment (FSA) using nine scales adapted from the Formal Elements Art Therapy Scale (FEATS). Unpublished paper.

Hammer, E. F. (1958). Expressive aspects of projective drawings. In E. F. Hammer (Ed.), *The clinical application of projective drawings* (6th ed., p. 59–79). Springfield, IL: Charles C Thomas.

Hammer, E. F. (1958). *The clinical application of projective drawings.* Springfield, IL: Charles C Thomas.

Hammer, E. F. (1975). *The clinical application of projective drawings* (4th ed.). Springfield, IL: Charles C Thomas.

Hammer, E. F. (1980). *The clinical application of projective drawings* (6th ed.). Springfield, IL: Charles C Thomas Publishing,

Horovitz-Darby, E. G. (1988). Art therapy assessment of a minimally language skilled deaf child. Proceedings from the 1988 University of California's Center on Deafness Conference: *Mental Health Assessment of Deaf Clients: Special Conditions,* Little Rock, AK: ADARA

Horovitz-Darby, E. G. (1991). Family art therapy within a deaf system. *Arts in Psychotherapy.* Vol. 18, 251–261.

Horovitz, E. G. (1985). A review of the silver drawing test of cognitive and creative skills. *Journal of Art Therapy,* March, (Vol. 2), 1:44.

Horovitz, E. (1995). *Art Therapy Program Textbook.* Rochester, NY: Nazareth College of Rochester.

Horovitz, E. G. (1999). *A leap of faith: The call to art.* (2nd ed.). Springfield, IL: Charles C Thomas.

Horovitz, E. G. (2002). *Spiritual art therapy: An alternate path* (2nd ed.). Springfield, IL: Charles C Thomas.

Horovitz, E. G. (2002). *Art Therapy and Speech/Language Therapy: An Interdisciplinary Approach.* [DVD]. Rochester, NY: Julia Production, 16-minute film.

Horovitz, E. G. (2006). Personal communication.

Horovitz, E. G. (2005). *Art therapy as witness: A sacred guide.* Springfield, IL: Charles C Thomas.

Horovitz, E. (2007, September 5th). Tables of comparative norms. Message posted to http://nazareth.blackboard.com/webapps/portal/frameset.jsp?tab=courses&url=/bin/co mmon/course.pl?course_id=_45204_1.

Horovitz, E. G. (Ed.). (2007). *Visually speaking: Art therapy and the deaf.* Springfield, IL: Charles C Thomas.

Horovitz, E. G. (2008). Personal Communications.

Horovitz, E. G., & Schulze, W. D. (2008). Society for the Arts in Healthcare, 19th Annual Conference Philadelphia, PA; Art Therapy & Stroke: New research on mood and stress reduction, April 18, 2008.

Hulse, W. C. (1951). The emotionally disturbed child draws his family. *Family. Quart. J. Child Behavior,* 3:152–174.

Hulse, W. C. (1952). Child conflict expressed through drawings. *Journal of Allergy and Clinical Immunology.* 16: 66–79.

Jung, C. G. (1965). *Memories, dreams, and reflections.* New York: Vintage Books.

Kast, V. (1992). *The dynamics of symbols: Fundamentals of Jungian psychotherapy.* New York, NY: Fromm International.

Koppitz, E. (1968). *The Bender-Gestalt test for young children.* New York, NY: Grune & Stratton, Inc.

Kramer, E. (2001). Sublimation and Art Therapy. In J. Ruben (Ed.), *Approaches to art therapy: Theory and technique* (2nd ed., p. 29–39). New York, NY: Brunner-Rutledge.

Levy, S. (1950). Figure drawing as a projective test. In Abt, L. & Bellak, L. (Eds.), *Projective psychology* (p. 257–279). New York: Knopf.

Levy, S., & Levy, R. A. (1958). Symbolism in animal drawings. In E. F. Hammer (Ed.), *The clinical application of projective drawings* (6th ed., p. 311–343). Springfield, IL: Charles C Thomas.

Lowenfeld, V. (1939). *The nature of creativity.* New York, NY: Harcourt, Brace.

Lowenfeld, V. (1947). *Creative and mental growth.* New York, NY: Macmillan.

Lowenfeld & Brittain. *Stages: Summary chart.* Lorette Wilmot Library PDF file.

Lowenfeld, V., & Brittain, W. L. (1975). *Creative and mental growth.* NY: MacMillan.

Lowenfeld, V., & Brittain, W. L. (1985). *Creative and mental growth* (6th ed.). New York: Macmillan.

Lowenfeld, V., & Brittain, W. L. (1987). *Creative and mental growth.* New York: Macmillan.

Machover, K. (1949). *Personality projection in the drawing of the human figure.* Springfield, IL: Charles C Thomas.

Malchiodi, C. (2003). *Handbook of art therapy.* New York, NY: The Guilford Press.

McGoldrick, M., Gerson, R., & Petry, S. (2008). *Genograms: Assessment and intervention* (3rd Edition). New York, NY: W.W. Norton & Company.

Misra, T., Connolly, A. M., & Majeed, A. (2006). Addressing mental health needs of asylum seekers and refugees in a London Borough: Epidemiological and user perspectives. *Primary Health Care Research and Development, 7,* 241–248.

Oster, G. D., & Crone, P. G. (2004). *Using drawings in assessment and therapy* (2nd ed.). New York, NY: Brunner-Routledge.

Peck, M. S. (1983). *People of the lie: The hope for healing human evil.* New York: Simon and Schuster.

Piaget, J. (1970). *Genetic epistemology.* New York: Columbia Press.

Piotrowski, C. (1995). A review of the clinical and research use of the Bender-Gestalt Test. *Perceptual and Motor Skills, 81,* 1272–1274.

Rasch, G. (1960). *Probabilistic models for some intelligence and attainment tests.* Copenhagen, Denmark: Danmarks Paedagogiske Institut.

Rivière, P. A. (1950). El juega de construir casas:su interpretation ye su valor diagnostico. *Rev. psicolanal,* 7:347–388.

Robb, M. (2001). Beyond the orphanages: Art therapy with Russian children. *Art Therapy: Journal of the American Art Therapy Association, 19* (4), 146–150.

Savin, D., Seymour, D., Littleford, L. N., & Giese, A., (2005). Findings from mental health screening of newly arrived refugees in Colorado. *Public Health Reports,* 120: 224–229.

Silver, R. (2002). *Three Art Assessments: The Silver Drawing Test of cognition and emotion; Draw a story: Screening for depression; and stimulus drawings and techniques.* New York, NY: Brunner-Routledge.

Stevenson, D. B. (1992). *Freud's psychosexual stages of development,* from http://www.victorian web.org/science/freud/develop.html.

Swan-Foster, N., Foster, S., & Dorsey, A. (2003). The use of the human figure drawing during pregnancy. *Journal of Reproductive and Infant Psychology, Volume 21,* Number 4, pp. 297–307.

Withrow, R. L. (2004). The Use of Color in Art Therapy. *Journal of Humanistic Counseling, Education and Development, 43,* 33–40.

Young in Art: The age of symbolism. http://www.arts.ufl.edu/art/rt_room/teach/young_in_art/sequence/symbolism.html.

AUTHOR INDEX

A

Albertson, J., vii, xiv, 177, 178
Anschela, D. J., 78, 297
Ashbrook, J. B., 26, 297
Atkinson, J. M., vii, 6, 58, 148, 166, 225

B

Bender, L., 39, 297
Betts, D. J., vii, xiii, 77, 78, 82, 84, 146, 297, 298
Brannigan, G. C., 40, 42, 45, 47, 297
Brittain, W. L., xiii, 17, 21, 29, 30, 38, 50, 57, 58, 60, 62, 69, 72, 73, 75, 76, 129, 131, 148, 172, 195, 204, 205, 214, 255, 268, 269, 299
Brooke, S. L., 90, 297
Buck, J. N., 86, 297
Burns, R. C., xiii, 22, 75, 125, 131, 132, 135, 136, 138, 180, 191, 192, 297
Butcher, D., vii, viii, 94, 229

C

Cheyne-King, S. E., 30, 80, 297
Cohen, F. W., 214, 297
Connolly, A. M., xiv, 177, 299
Crone, P., 20, 21, 65, 72, 135, 88, 90, 91, 93, 94, 96, 99, 101, 102, 104, 106, 128, 129, 136, 148, 162, 171, 172, 184, 185, 186, 187, 192, 214, 251, 299

D

Dearing, T., 24, 297

D

Decker, S. L., 40, 42, 45, 47, 297
DeRoller, J., viii, 45, 230
DiLeo, J. H., 125, 297
Dombeck, M., 24, 25, 297
Dorsey, A., 78, 300

E

Eksten, S. L., viii, xii, 8, 19, 127, 170, 233

F

Foster, S., 78, 300
Fowler, J. W., 29, 36, 195, 297
Frank, J. B., 24, 297
Frank, J. D., 24, 297

G

Gantt, L., xiv, 22, 78, 143, 144, 145, 146, 148, 155, 156, 162, 192, 298
Gerson, R., 4, 299
Giese, A., xiv, 177, 299
Griffiths, R., 86, 298
Guerin, P., 26, 298

H

Hall, J., 30, 298
Hamilton, M., 77, 78, 298
Hammer, E. F., xiii, 20, 21, 22, 23, 29, 35, 36, 58, 60, 64, 65, 70, 72, 75, 80, 86, 87, 88, 90, 93, 94, 96, 99, 100, 101, 102, 103, 104, 105, 106, 125, 129, 135, 148, 154, 155, 156, 162, 171, 182, 184, 185, 192, 214, 298, 299

301

SUBJECT INDEX

A

achromatic, xxii, xxiii, 89, 91, 92, 93, 94, 96, 97, 98, 99, 100, 101, 102, 103, 104, 105, 106, 107, 108, 146, 182, 184, 185, 186, 229
Adolescent Art, 268
Adult Stage, 29, 182, 195, 268
Africa, vii, viii, xi, xiv, xix, 177, 178, 179, 181, 182, 183, 184, 185, 186, 187, 189, 191, 192, 193, 195, 197
aggression, 20, 42, 60, 96, 101, 106, 128, 135, 189
American Sign Language (ASL), 201, 203, 208, 278, 279
Anal Stage, 17, 18, 22, 147, 298
anxiety, 16, 18, 36, 42, 48, 57, 68, 69, 70, 71, 75, 76, 84, 85, 88, 93, 128, 135, 136, 147, 155, 162, 180, 228, 232, 240, 249, 253
Art Therapy Dream Assessment (ATDA), xii, xix, xxi, xxv, 8, 13, 15, 16, 17, 19, 22, 28, 88, 109, 127, 129, 146, 154, 170, 172, 223, 233, 239
Artistic Stage, 18, 146, 147, 182, 195, 269
autism, 77

B

Belief Art Therapy Assessment (BATA), xii, xix, xxi, xxiii, xxv, xxvi, 22, 24, 25, 26, 27, 28, 30, 31, 32, 33, 34, 35, 36, 37, 38, 79, 109, 110, 123, 154, 173, 178, 193, 194, 195, 239, 241, 251, 270, 278
Bender-Gestalt II, xiii, xv, xix, xxi, 39, 40, 41, 42, 43, 44, 45, 46, 47, 48, 49, 227, 230, 297
Brain Injured Stage, 50, 269

C

Catholic, 29, 36, 193, 196, 240, 248, 249, 251, 284, 286, 288
Christianity, 193, 196
chromatic, xxii, xxiii, xxv, 87, 88, 89, 90, 91, 92, 94, 95, 96, 97, 98, 99, 100, 101, 102, 103, 104, 105, 106, 116, 117, 118, 119, 120, 146, 182, 184, 185, 186, 229
Cognitive Art Therapy Assessment (CATA), xiii, xv, xix, xxi, xxii, xxiii, xxv, xxvi, 6, 38, 50, 57, 58, 59, 61, 62, 63, 64, 65, 67, 68, 69, 71, 73, 74, 75, 76, 82, 85, 107, 110, 111, 112, 122, 134, 136, 148, 161, 162, 166, 178, 179, 180, 181, 183, 195, 203, 204, 205, 225, 237, 243, 248, 270, 295
compartmentalization, xiii, 125, 136
Crayola^{c}, 77, 87

D

Deaf, vii, viii, 6, 7, 50, 200, 201, 203, 204, 225, 226, 280, 284, 291, 298
deaf, 50, 298
Diagnostic Drawing Series (DDS), 30, 278
Drawing from Imagination, xxiii, 164, 165, 166, 169, 170, 173, 176, 190
Drawing from Observation, xxiii, 165, 166, 168, 173, 175, 187, 189
DSM-IV, xii, 3, 146, 278

E

Eosinophilic Gastroenteritis (EG), 6, 7, 225, 226

303